The **Code**

of

Life

The Anti-Aging, Disease Prevention, and
Recovery Breakthrough of our Lifetime!!

Dr. Ronald P. Drucker (B.S., M.T.A.S.C.P.), D.C.
Dr. Sergey Sorin, M.D.

Printed in the United States of America.

Copyright© 2020
Washington D.C Library Of Congress #1-9120187921

For purposes of simplicity and ease, this book; The Code of Life, The Anti-Aging, Disease Prevention and Recovery Breakthrough of our Lifetime, will henceforth be referred to as *"The Code of Life..."*

The wonderful news about to be shared, can and will change your life forever. In all probability, it will also extend your life if you take it to heart and take simple action.

Many scientists studying mortality now believe that aging is really a "dis-ease," and not the inevitable experience of the biological organism.

Aging and disease are not our predetermined fate, but instead they are the fate that we have been taught to assume by those who deceive us.

This book opens the eyes of the reader in numerous ways which dramatically affect life and our very existence. Things that we have been led to believe by those we may trust are revealed, to our amazement, to be no less than clever fabrications of reality.

Although shocking and somewhat disturbing at times, in the end the information contained within is ultimately the most joyous and liberating news we could possibly receive as human beings.

It is the answer we have all been waiting for!

The Authors:

Dr. Ronald P. Drucker, (B.S., M.T.A.S.C.P.), D.C.

Dr. Sergey Sorin, M.D., Medical Director of The World Famous Shealy/Sorin Wellness Institute.

With over sixty-five combined years experience in research, formulation, natural healing techniques, therapies, and most importantly, repeated success against "incurable" chronic autoimmune and degenerative diseases, Dr. Drucker and Dr. Sorin are known among their colleagues and patients as among the very best in the field of healing.

"There could be no greater a heinous crime, than the premeditated withholding of truth from the masses, to the point of their injury or death."

Having a life-long interest and passion for healing, and after dedicating our lives to the study and practice of the healing arts, We have written this book on the single most significant discovery relating to health; the discovery of **The Code of Life**, *in relation to cellular communication, what it means to man-kind, and why those in power want it silenced.*

"Each progressive spirit is opposed by a thousand mediocre minds appointed to guard the past."

-- Maurice Maeterlinck

Dedication

To all those seeking better health,
and a longer, higher quality of life.

To the healthy and ill, privileged and impoverished
alike trapped within the system,
and to all those who have lost the quality of
life, or even life itself, to the detriment of missing,
withheld, or misleading information.

To our family, friends, and colleagues,
whose constant support has
made this publication possible…
…we are eternally grateful.

To all, we wish great health, long life, and
exceptional living all along the way.

An Eternal Thanks to Amanda, whose perseverance, unending
aid, and attention to detail made this entire process possible.
"I can no other answer make, but, thanks, and thanks."
~William Shakespeare

A Special Thanks to Kathryn, our establishment insider
and friend, who through endless hours of research provided
many of the of the medical statistics throughout this book.

A Very Special Thanks to Meriruth,
for all which may go unsaid.

Contents

Dedication   7

Foreword   11
The Ultimate Conflict of Interest   12
Is it *"Healthcare"* or "Disease Care"?   12
The Basic Health Facts...   14

Overview   17
Against the Design   17
The Human Design   17
Failure by Design   18
Perfect Fuel and Medicine by Design   20
Damaging and Misleading Terminology   27
How did the term *"side effects"* come about?   31
Pay no attention to the man behind the curtain!   32
Symptom Relief Roulette (SRR)   33
The Tricks of the Trade   34

Introduction
An Argument in the Industry   37
Understanding the Cure   40
Who's in Charge?   45

A Note to the Reader   50

Chapter 1
The Code, The Spectrum,* and *The Symphony of Life   52
The Keys to Health, Youth, and Longevity   52
A Synthetic *"Vitamin"* is not a Vitamin   55
The Body is a Whole   58
Perfect Cellular Support   59
Healthy Digestion: The Masked Doorway to Health, Disease
Prevention, and Recovery.   59
Some Very Good News   60

The average healing time frames reported for The Most   62
Common Autoimmune Conditions
Common Autoimmune Symptoms List   67

The COVID-19 Charade   70
It is more than Wise to Armor Oneself   72

Where do these Immune Modulating Components come from?   74

Chapter 2
Anti-Aging and Cell Regeneration   75

Science has discovered that vital nutrients regulate
RNA/DNA Gene Expression and Cell Life Span!   76
"The Cell is Immortal"   79
How to effectively combat aging and disease, *simplified*   80
The Alkaline Environment   81
Addressing Stress   83

Chapter 3
The Code of Life
Cellular Communication   86
A Perspective on "Disease"   87
Second Note to the Reader   90
Tracking Down the Code   91
The Miracle Plant   94

Chapter 4
What Has Happened To Our Food?   98
Overeating Yet Under-Feeding   103
Essential Co-Factors   105
The *Slow* Death List   107
Food Recommendations for Optimum Health
Beauty Without Substance   109
"Certified Organic"   110
"Food Pyramids" - both hopeless and impossible guidelines   114
Phytonutrient Supplementation   115
Take Your Cod Liver Oil!   116
Nutritional Protocol for Prevention, Anti-Aging, and
  Disease Recovery   117
The Common Fruits and Vegetables List   119
Here Comes the Sun   119

Chapter 5
The Current State of Modern Medicine
Schizo-Care U.S.A.   122
Drugs Gone Wild!   125
The Biological Terrain   129
"Always Searching for The Cures," …   132
  but where are the cures?

An Attitude Revealed   135
Critical Health Information Withheld or Inaccurate   136

What's the Mystery?   141
The Invasion of The Health Snatchers   142
What's in *Your* Wallet?   142

Technical (Chapters 6, 7 & 8)
Chapter 6
The Amazing Immune System   144

Chapter 7
The Functions of the Carbohydrates making up
   the Symbols of The Code   150
The Glycocalyx, or *"The Fuzz"*   151
The Biochemistry of Cellular Communication   152
Special Receptors Lying in Wait   154
Intracellular Communication   156
The Process of Exocytosis   157
Other Important Functions of the Essential Carbohydrates   159
The Difference Between Simple and Complex Sugars   162

Chapter 8
The Critical Nature of Proper Digestion and the
   Role of the Complex Carbohydrate   167
The Protectors   169
The Communicators   171
The Miracle of Endocytosis   172
Probiotics and the Polysaccharides   173

Conclusion   177
THE HIPPOCRATIC OATH   181
References   182

Foreword

How much is truly known about longevity? Does our government really want all of us to live one hundred healthy years and beyond? Has the anti-aging secret been uncovered and then concealed in the name of power, profit, and control?

Human-kind already possesses the knowledge to live a long, healthy, disease-free existence. *The answer* has been withheld from us. The preventions and cures for the majority of diseases are known, and the astounding fact is, they are not *complex* as we have been led to believe . . . most are one and the same.

It is an undisputed scientific fact that disease prevention, health, healing, beauty, and anti-aging all begin at the cellular level. The health of your cells dictates the health of your body, *and* your mind. WE ARE CELLS! Trillions of cells make up our bodies. Every tissue, organ, gland, cartilage, bone, muscle, and nerve, which amounts to every single part of our bodies are made up of cells.

Authors, Dr. Ronald P. Drucker and Sergey Sorin, M.D. reveal to us that in most cases, *"incurable diseases"* are not incurable at all, and our *"modern medical system"* is not providing us with solutions that have been recognized as fact by scientists for decades. The fact is, the cure for most diseases and the effective solution to prevention, health, healing, beauty, and anti-aging is already known and available.

The Fountain of Youth, *and Health*, is not located on some far away island. It is located within each and every one of our cells. It involves perfect cellular health, unrestricted cellular communication, and subsequently, uninhibited/unaltered DNA replication. The language our cells utilize to communicate with each other and the immune system is *"The Code of Life."* Vital healing components are needed which metaphorically make up the *"symbols"* of this cellular language. Against the will of the pharmaceutical drug establishment, *it is all about to be revealed to you!*

The Ultimate Conflict of Interest

What is going on in our healthcare industry today? Are the large pharmaceutical corporations truly interested in finding cures for disease? Is the pharmaceutical industry, whose profits are based on large segments of the population suffering from major illnesses, interested in eliminating their customer base? We can tell you from over sixty-five combined years experience in healthcare, including thirty-five combined years of hospital, clinical laboratory, and medical research projects, that the answer is a resounding... NO!

As physicians using natural means to treat our patients, we have been able to focus our attention on natural and safe alternatives to drugs. The economically lucrative drugs that are approved by the FDA (Food and Drug Administration) at enormous expense, and many of which are eventually pulled off the market due to adverse reactions, are designed to alleviate symptoms, but rarely if ever address the cause of the disease.

Is it *"Healthcare"* or Disease Care?

True *"healthcare"* would be the care of the very basic unit of life, which as we know is the human cell. This comprehensive care would begin in our very early years, conceivably from conception, involving a system focused on the healthy maintenance of the cells and thus, the non-interference of cellular function and subsequently unaltered DNA replication. This effective healthcare system would begin before we were born with our pregnant mothers commencing a comprehensive regimen of specific nutrient-targeting to ensure the optimal cellular development of a healthy newborn infant.

What has just been described in the last paragraph could be summed up with the term prevention. Real healthcare implies prevention. As we know, there is no such mainstream medicine system regimen focused from conception, or at any time for that matter, specifically on the health of our cells. Therefore, there is no specific system of prevention within mainstream medicine and subsequently the use of the term *"healthcare"* as used by the current establishment is completely inaccurate and misleading.

So, what is the system currently in use designed to accomplish? For example, when we experience an ache or pain to the point that it becomes bothersome or unbearable, we make an appointment with our doctor to have a *"let's see."* Our doctor attempts to diagnose (an industry estimated 50% of the time with accuracy) our condition through testing and the various clues of our symptoms. He or she then most often prescribes a pharmaceutical medication designed to address the symptoms. Fifty percent of the time it will be the drug *approved* for the condition. In the overwhelming majority of cases, only the symptoms will be addressed, not the underlying condition or its cause, and in doing so the *symptoms* of the disease will be *managed* at best while the disease itself progresses. Would the term *"disease care"* best describe this system? If this correct and accurate term were used to describe this system, no one would partake in the system. No one would be interested in *"disease care."* No one would purchase *"disease insurance."* No one would be interested in *"maintaining their disease."*

In order to market a system to the public whose underlying motivation is the sale of economically lucrative drugs and medical procedures, one must create false atmospheres via the use of soft terms. *"Healthcare"* and perfect health are what we are all seeking, but this is not what the system is structured to deliver. The problem with the current system is that *caring for disease* is very profitable, while *preventing disease* is not. The structure of the entire system is a financial conflict-of-interest in which the patient most often pays with their time, money, health, and eventually their lives.

The drug industry contributes heavily to political campaigns which places tremendous pressure on our "representatives" to maintain the status quo of The System. The medical and pharmaceutical industries are the benefactors of illness in America. These are the industries that thrive on the economics of disease. This is the modern-day *Cartel*.

The simplicity of optimal health and disease prevention through the specific support of cellular requirements is the hidden truth which their curtain conceals from public understanding.

In order to effectively market their myriad of harmful concoctions, they must continue to convince us that the health issues are complex. They have spent billions in their attempt to convince us of this complexity and for many decades they have been successful. They believe that the masses are ignorant and their smoke and mirror marketing tactics designed to lead the public away from the effective natural solution will be permitted to continue without exposure. They continue to urge us to *"ask our doctors about,"* their *"solutions,"* which for the most part are toxic chemicals designed to address the symptoms of the underlying health problems - in essence, problems which they, themselves, have created over decades through their campaign of misinformation. They have suppressed the basic truths of health.

The Basic Health Facts . . .

The Pharma/Medical Establishment does not want the public to understand these basic facts:

1. **Specific nutrient and phytonutrient deficiency (causing cellular starvation and subsequent DNA damage) is the primary factor involving premature aging and degenerative disease.**
2. **Specific nutrients, phytonutrients, and co-factors in adequate amounts are the prevention and cure to premature aging and most existing diseases.**

2. **An oxygen-rich, alkaline extracellular environment and the maintenance of the optimum biological terrain is an environment in which disease cannot thrive.**

3. **Profit-based synthetic drugs or compounds, and synthetic or artificial substances are not what the human body is designed to receive. The overwhelming majority of these substances cause short and long term cellular damage to varying degrees, without addressing the root causes of disease.**

Having a life-long interests and passions for healing, and after dedicating our lives to the study and practice of the healing arts, we have written this book on the single most significant discovery relating to health; the understanding of the function and effect of specific nutritional components in relation to cellular support and communication, disease prevention, disease recovery, and effective anti-aging.

First and foremost, and against the will of *The Cartel*, the reader will be widely introduced to the phytonutrients, and in particular, natural polymannan molecules (immune modulators) and their diverse healing effects on the human body. These profound healing molecules have been referred to by scientists as *"Healing Orchestrators"* or *"Conductor Molecules."* These, in conjunction with other specific nutrients and phytonutrients become the components which enable cells to communicate with other cells and with the immune system, to perform an entire array of health functions including; the elimination of foreign invaders such as viruses, harmful bacteria, and diseased cells. These special components of communication metaphorically make up the "symbols" of this physiological language. These are the symbols of *"The Code of Life"* representing a vast and complex physiological science of cells communicating with other cells within our bodies. The power of these molecules to bring astounding benefit to the suffering public is understood by many scientists, and yet in today's pharmaceutically controlled medical culture, the good news has found little public forum until now.

Secondly and equally as important, the reader will be widely informed of the fact that these molecules and healing components, along with specific nutrients all taken in adequate quantities are indeed the prevention and cure for most diseases known to man. They are also the most efficient and effective general health, weight control, beauty and anti-aging solution due to the proven fact that they promote the proper functioning of the human cell, as designed!

We want to emphasize the importance of reading the findings and health benefits listed in this book. In order to form a solid habit in regard to ingesting the vital nutrients daily, we must be consciously aware of the multitude of health benefits we are gaining. This awareness provides strong motivation to form the needed habit, and thus reap the health and longevity rewards. If we are ingesting specific nutrients because we heard they are *"The Code of Life,"* but we do not really understand most or all of the benefits, we may lose focus. The most important thing to remember about fighting and preventing aging and disease through nutritional cellular support, is that it should be done consistently every day. Obviously eating good quality food, swallowing a few capsules, or taking some nutrient powder with juice is a small price to pay for quality-of-life and longevity. More good news is that depending on your present and ongoing level of health, after healing you will be able to taper off the quantity ingested and still receive adequate cellular support.

Overview

Against the Design

We all understand what would happen if we put gasoline into the fuel tank of a car with a diesel engine, or vice versa. Needless to say, damage would occur to the engines of both vehicles because we attempted to use a source of energy for which the engines were not designed. The damage would occur quickly and be immediately apparent. Two damaging processes would take place. In both cases, the engines would be starved for the components they need to operate smoothly, while being damaged by components they are not designed for.

Another example would be if we were to attempt to run a high performance engine on 87 octane gasoline, which demands 94 octane by design. In this case, the damage would be less noticeable, but would occur over time until the engine was prematurely destroyed. The engine would experience damage and ultimately fail because the fuel utilized was "low-grade" or "inadequate" to meet the demands of the engine's functions and design.

The Human Design

Although many of us are not familiar with the internal workings of a combustion engine and may think of it as complex, in reality it is a crude and simplistic invention in comparison to the intricate design of the human body and in particular, the human cell. The examples relating to engines, fuels, and designs above are elementary and easy for all of us to understand because inherently we know what happens when we go against *"The Laws of Design."* As you read on you may be wondering how we as a society have been convinced that we can get away with going against the *laws of design* in regard to what we put into our bodies. The answer is *premeditated ill-design* in the form of clever, misleading and deceptive marketing by an industry whose profits are generated by illness, not health or healing. (more on this to follow).

The human cell, the very foundation of human life, possesses an intricate and highly sophisticated design. Individual cells are invisible to the naked eye and yet a multitude of processes occur within them dictating our health, appearance, quality of life and ultimately our lifespan. The cell contains many components which perform an entire array of vital functions for the body. Within the nucleus of the cell, genetic material (DNA) is the chemical blueprint or master plan for the cell. The cell is the foundation of health and life. The cell has <u>specific requirements that must be constantly met</u> in order to avoid cellular starvation, deterioration, pre-mature aging and ultimately disease.

Most scientists and engineers agree that the human being is the most intricate and amazing design known to the planet. Whether you believe that the creator is "God" or "Nature," everyone agrees that the designer was not man. Man did not design or create man. Man did not design or create the earth or the universe. Man, regardless of desire or ego, does not possess the knowledge to fully comprehend the complexity of nature or the human blueprint. With each new scientific discovery concerning the human body we are yet further amazed by the majesty and intricacy of this grand design, obviously conceived by an intelligence far superior to our own.

All the necessary components and nutrients for the sustenance of human life, as well as all living creatures on the planet, were also designed by this *Superior Intelligence*, not by man.

Failure by Design

The current Periodic Table of Elements used universally in the field of chemistry lists 110 known elements including; gases, solids, liquids and "synthetics." Twenty out of the 110 known elements listed are man-made or synthetic. Reflective of man's ability to create a *"superior"* element is the fact that ALL TWENTY man-made synthetic elements are either a contamination hazard, radioactive, or both!

A wise person concedes the fact, that for man to claim the ability to create a *"superior"* design opposed to the natural food sources and healing agents of the *Superior Intelligence,* for the long-term benefit of man is simply misguided falsehoods and foolish arrogance motivated in large by lust for profit.

Many things are marketed to us to ensure profits. Products for internal consumption such as foods, pharmaceuticals and even some nutritional supplements are made to appear attractive or beneficial. In most instances, they are not what the human body is designed to receive. Organic/Natural is the design for humans. Humans are not designed for *synthetics.* They *are not* what we are designed for. Synthetics are the wrong fuel or energy source for the human body design. Damage inevitably occurs, short and long term when we attempt to replace natural with most synthetics.

There is an old, well known cliché; *"Throw a monkey wrench into the machinery."* It originated from mechanics that would occasionally lose their grip on a tool such as a monkey wrench. The wrench would fall into a running engine, getting caught in moving parts, causing damage. The cliché infers that if you throw something into a system that does not belong there, you may cause damage or destroy the entire system.

We refer to synthetics, whether drugs or synthetic supplements as *"Biological Monkey-Wrenches."* When we introduce these unnatural substances into our bodies, we induce stress upon our entire system until these substances can be eliminated. The cellular damage caused by unnatural, against-the-design substances varies widely from reversible to lethal and all levels of damage in between.

Many drugs manufactured are originally derived from a natural compound found in nature. Through synthetic molecular alteration, the patentable drug is created. Nearly all drugs have unwanted *"side effects,"* which are in reality, <u>*direct unwanted effects upon the body.*</u> These unwanted effects occur due to this unnatural alteration of nature's original chemical profiles. <u>Natural substances cannot be patented</u>. The pharmaceutical industry attempts to market the impression that their patent-for-profit, synthetic molecular alterations are somehow *"superior"* or *"advanced"* in comparison to the healing agents found in nature, created by The Superior Intelligence. In a sublime manner they attempt to convince us that The Superior Intelligence does not know what is best for us.

Common sense tells us that in order for a treatment to be superior, or even compatible with the human body, it would need to benefit all areas, or specific areas of the body without causing harm to any other area or areas. The presence of these direct unwanted or harmful effects is proof positive that man has failed to accomplish this task. It is rather some men, who do not know what is best for us, or who are simply unwilling to acknowledge fact for reasons of financial gain.

When given some serious thought, is it not amazing and **infuriating** that Big Pharma would have the audacity to attempt to frighten the public away from many of the side-effect-free healing compounds found in nature, some of the very compounds used as the basis of their synthetic drugs and products prior to molecular alteration?

Perfect Fuel and Medicine by Design

The perfect human fuels and medicines come from plant-derived foods and are referred to as *Phytonutrients.* The term *phytonutrient,* (plant-nutrient), is derived from the Greek word *phyto,* meaning plant, and *nutrient;* a constituent of food, vital for physiological function. A phytonutrient is a plant-derived natural nutrient. Phytonutrients are biologically active compounds in plant-derived foods that elicit biological activity throughout the body.

There are numerous classes of phytonutrients, many of which can contain scores of different phytonutrients. Many overlaps and complement one another working synergistically to boost total health benefits. We estimate that upwards of 1,000 phytonutrients have been identified to date and many more of these remain yet undiscovered. Some of the more vital forms, many not seen listed on government websites or literature, or *classified* as phytonutrients are; ajoenes, allylic sulfides, amino acids, anthocyanins, anti-oxidants, betaines, bioflavinoids, capsaicin, carotenoids, catechins, chelating agents, chlorophyll, complex carbohydrates, coumarins, cyclic compounds, enzymes, essential fatty acids, flavonoids, flavonols, flavones, flavanones, gamma-oryzanol glucomannans, glucopolymannans, hydroxycinnamic acids, isoflavones, isothiocyanates, indoles, lignans, limonoids, mannans, methionine reductase, mucopolysaccharides, organic minerals, organic trace minerals, organic vitamins, phenols, phospholipids, phytosterols, polymannans, polyphenols, polysaccharides, plant proteins, resveratrol, saponins, sulfides, thiols, terpenes, and tocopherols to name just a few. Some of those mentioned above are classes, others are subclasses.

<u>Researchers are finding that the same phytonutrients that keep plants free from disease also perform the very same function within our bodies.</u> The list of health benefits is virtually endless and includes cellular fueling and repair, increasing cell life (anti-aging), the inhibition of cancer-producing substances and the prevention of degenerative diseases to name just a few. In short, specific phytonutrients found in certain fruits, vegetables and the plants themselves, work synergistically to protect our health.

Science has proven the effectiveness of this perfect natural human *fuel and medicine* through countless studies to date. What would we expect to find, concerning the fuel and medicine designed for the human, by the creator of the human?

Drug industry misinformation is generated in multiple forms in the attempt to disguise and down-play these scientific facts; one of the most obvious being the misuse of the name *phytonutrient* itself. If millions of people were not dying (made and kept ill), due to *The Pharmaceutical Cartel*-generated confusion, their attempts of disguising the obvious would almost be amusing.

Despite political and financial pressures placed upon the various government agencies to down-play and disguise these facts, due to the magnitude of the subject (public health, life, and death), they must publish them *somewhere* so that they themselves are *covered.* Let us examine the way it is done.

The United States Department of Agriculture (USDA); Quote:

"The term "phyto" originated from a Greek word meaning plant. Phytonutrients are certain organic components of plants, and these components are thought to promote human health. Fruits, vegetables,

grains, legumes, nuts and teas are rich sources of phytonutrients. Unlike the traditional nutrients (protein, fat, vitamins, minerals), phytonutrients are not "essential" for life, so some people prefer the term "phytochemical".

One could have a field-day with this paragraph alone. Compare it to the first paragraph in this section. Notice that in defining the word phytonutrient for the suffering public, somehow, they failed to define the word nutrient.

Here are three common definitions of the word **nutrient:**

1. A constituent of food, vital for physiological function.
2. Any substance that can be metabolized by an organism to give energy and build tissue.
3. A chemical element or compound used in an organism's metabolism or physiology.

Obviously, each definition of the word nutrient indicates that it is a substance <u>vital for physiological function</u>, or **Life**.

Now look at the third sentence in the USDA's paragraph;

"Unlike the traditional nutrients (protein, fat, vitamins, minerals), phytonutrients are not "essential" for life, so some people prefer the term "phytochemical"

First and foremost, when you see the word *"traditional,"* used in this context, you can justifiably suspect that the current "traditional" Pharma/Medical Establishment may be largely responsible for the classification.

Secondly, why would *"some people"* who *somehow* forgot to define the word *nutrient,* for the suffering public, define phytonutrients as not *"essential"* for life?

In addition, why would *"some people"* prefer to use the term *"phytochemical,"* when most know that even though everything on earth is *"chemical,"* the word *chemical* frightens a majority of the public away from consumption?

Could *"some people"* be the pharmaceutical industry and/ or those who do their bidding?

There is one more interesting reason why they must keep the term *phytonutrients* separate from *"traditional nutrients"* such as *vitamins and minerals* . . . because the overwhelming majority of *"vitamins and minerals"* on the market today are synthetic and not plant-derived at all (see more about this on page 55). The pharmaceutical industry is also responsible for the manufacturing of many of these synthetics as well.

For now, let us have a look at the various statements below. Although these government statements are purposely worded *mildly* as to not interfere too much with big-business, let us decide for ourselves if phytonutrients are *"non-essential"* for our lives or the lives of our loved ones.

Centers for Disease Control and Prevention: *"Current evidence collectively demonstrates that fruit and vegetable intake is associated with improved health, reduced risk of major diseases, and possibly delayed onset of age-related factors."*

The World Cancer Research Fund and the American Institute for Cancer Research: *"Evidence of dietary protection against cancer is strongest and most consistent for diets high in vegetables and fruits."*

Food and drug Administration (FDA): *"Diets rich in fruits and vegetables may reduce the risk of some types of cancer and other chronic diseases."*

The United States Department of Agriculture (USDA): *"While these phytonutrients aren't "essential" by traditional definitions, they apparently reduce risks of diseases of aging."*

USDA: "Phytonutrients Take Center Stage"; *"Now there's a new surge of discovery around health-enhancing compounds in plant foods known as phytonutrients."*

USDA: *"Indeed, cancer, heart disease, and Alzheimer's disease may plague the middle-aged and elderly because of our limited knowledge of phytonutrients"* . . . *"Certain flavonoids in blueberries may actually reverse nerve cell aging. And a wide array of compounds in fruits and vegetables may protect cell components against oxidative damage as well as vitamins C or E."*

USDA: *"Plant foods contain biologically active components beyond those defined as essential nutrients, such as thousands of anti-oxidant phytochemicals that impart health benefits beyond the basic nutrition for an intended population."*

International Food Information Council (IFIC): *"Plant foods, such as fruits, vegetables, and whole grains contain many components that are beneficial to human health. Research supports that some of these foods, as part of an overall healthful diet, have the potential to delay the onset of many age-related diseases."*

IFIC: *"A recent review of current literature suggests that fruits and vegetables in combination have synergistic effects on antioxidant activities leading to greater reduction in risk of chronic disease, specifically for cancer and heart disease.*

IFIC: *"Most research indicates that there are overall health benefits from antioxidant-rich foods consumed in the diet."*

IFIC: *"Reinforced by current research, the message remains that antioxidants obtained from food sources, including fruits, vegetables, and whole grains, are potentially active in disease risk reduction and can be beneficial to human health."*

IFIC: *"Antioxidants, by their very nature, are capable of stabilizing free radicals before they can react and cause harm, in much the same way that a buffer stabilizes an acid to maintain a normal pH. Because oxidation is a naturally occurring process within the body, a balance with antioxidants must exist to maintain health."*

IFIC: *"An increasing body of evidence suggests beneficial effects of the antioxidants present in grapes, cocoa, blueberries, and teas on* *cardiovascular health, Alzheimer's disease, and even reduction of the risk of some cancers."*

Ohio State University, Family and Consumer Sciences: *"Although phytochemicals are not yet classified as nutrients, substances necessary for sustaining life, they have been identified as containing properties for aiding in disease prevention. Phytochemicals are associated with the prevention and/or treatment of at least four of the leading causes of death in the United States -- cancer, diabetes, cardiovascular disease, and hypertension. They are involved in many processes including ones that help prevent cell damage, prevent cancer cell replication, and decrease cholesterol levels."*

The published statements regarding the benefits of phytonutrients could fill this book, therefore, we will stop here.

For the benefit of our health, let us now intelligently define the term *phytonutrients:*

A phytonutrient is a plant-derived, biologically-active natural nutrient, essential and vital for optimum health, longevity, physiological function, and the prevention of diseases. They include all those mentioned in the second paragraph of this section, and so many more. Additionally, since plant **derived natural** vitamins, minerals, amino acids, complex carbohydrates, enzymes, co-factors, etc., are also plant-derived nutrients, this should place them in the *phytonutrient* (plant nutrient) category as well. All of them are phytonutrients, all prevent disease and/or promote health, and therefore, all are *essential.* A synthetic of any kind is *not* a phytonutrient. Should this be widely understood, it would *End* The Manufactured Confusion.

It is almost numbing to think that Big Pharma's deceptive marketing of their *"cure image"* over the last hundred years has been so effective that anyone, scientist or lay person, would be *surprised* to learn that the preventions and the cures for diseases are in the plants.

Natural or "organic" vitamins, minerals and nutrients are of biological origin. They are plant-derived nutrients (phytonutrients). In other words, they originate from a natural plant source. The plant's root hairs pull *inorganic* nutrients and minerals (the non-digestible form) from the water and soil, and through a chemical process involving photosynthesis, they are combined with organic molecules within the plant to form the organically bound nutrients. This is the form of food and medicine that we have been designed to utilize.

Why is the plant designed to extract inorganic earth minerals and nutrients from the soil and convert them to organically bound phytonutrients? The plant is preparing the nutrient in an absorbable form for consumption by another life form such as humans or animals.

Amazing, is it not? A plant is a "living machine" of sorts, designed by a Supreme Intelligence to provide absorbable and digestible "living nutrition" to sustain us, and natural medicines to protect and heal us. Has a plant ever been described to you in this manner? This is one function of a *food bearing* plant. Providing oxygen for us to breath is another.

Herein lies the modern-age dilemma: If the mineral or nutrient is no longer in the soil, it cannot be in the plant. This means that those plant constituents or phytonutrients normally made from the inorganic soil matter, such as vitamins, enzymes, and co-factors, subsequently cannot be produced within the plant either.

Soil depletion, chemical contamination, and pre-mature harvesting *(green-harvesting)* are the culprits of our present day low-grade, low-nutrient food supplies. We are running on "87 octane" when our engines are designed to receive 94! The difference between the two numbers, 87 and 94 in our simple analogy does not seem vast; however, the difference between a nutrient poor food supply and adequate nutrition is the difference between prolonged cellular life and pre-mature cellular death.

Damaging and Misleading Terminology

Currently within the U.S. Government and current medical community, it is *"officially recognized"* that there are at least 40 individual nutrients that have been proven, without a doubt, to be essential for human life. However, history has shown us that millions die while waiting for *official recognition, most* often of the scientifically obvious.

Aside from man-made synthetic, radioactive, and inert elements; the universe is composed of approximately 77 naturally occurring atomic elements found within the Periodic Table of Elements used in chemistry. All of these elements are naturally present within the human body, and utilized if made available. They exist within all plant and animal life. They are found in the waters of the oceans, the soils of the land, and within the atmosphere we breathe. They are the components of life on this planet. They are the wonderful keys of health, by the *Grand Design* of The Superior Intelligence.

There are quite possibly thousands of naturally occurring phytonutrients found within an organic natural food supply, many yet to be discovered. These miraculous compounds include complex carbohydrates, amino acids, fatty acids, enzymes, vitamins, minerals, and an entire array of co-factors. Co-factors are substances that need to be present in addition to an enzyme for specific physiologic reactions to take place.

Our choices boil down to a stark simplicity. We can continue to deteriorate while limiting ourselves to the *"officially recognized"* nutrients, recognized by a hierarchal establishment whose financial-based incentive lies in the delay of recognition, or we can heed to the overwhelming scientific literature (and common sense) which repeatedly shows the benefits of these natural, powerful, yet harmless nutrients and thus benefit accordingly. Most would agree that suffering while waiting for more of the essential nutrients to be *"recognized"* by the medical-drug cartel, already understood by the scientific community, is not the logical answer to health.

As you will learn, there exists an entire multitude of nutrients scientifically shown to be beneficial to health and longevity. Therefore, the term essential should not be the guideline or goal, but rather the provision of an optimum supply of nutrients.

The intelligent course of action to obtain optimum health, is clearly the consumption of the widest possible spectrum of naturally occurring, side-effect-free nutrients and phytonutrients available, in their purest bio-available form.

The arrogant mentality which would ignore science and infer that these components of life are of no useful consequence because they are not yet *"officially recognized,"* is the same schizophrenic mentality, upon befuddlement of purpose, that implies *these things are useless if we do not fully understand them.* This is the mentality which infers that drugs are more beneficial than consistent, diverse, and quality nutrition. It is this dangerous and dictatorial mentality at the helm of *"health care"* that has driven us far into an age of rapidly compounding degenerative diseases.

There exist many other damaging terms as well, curiously inserted within the common health vocabulary which are clearly counterproductive to public well-being.

For example, an accepted definition of an "essential nutrient" is; *a nutrient required for normal body functioning that cannot be synthesized by the body and must be obtained from a dietary source.* This is true, yet government agencies currently list approximately forty, while scientists have discovered and continue to discover hundreds, if not thousands of natural occurring life enhancing nutrients.

The *accepted* definition of a so-called *"non-essential nutrient"* is one that can be synthesized by the cell if absent from the food. In other words, under ideal circumstances the body can produce it, assuming there are adequate levels of the *"essential nutrients,"* enzymes, and co-factors necessary for its production. In today's world of nutrient-poor foods, this is assuming a great deal. Both these classifications have been accepted and perpetuated by the Pharmaceutical/Medical Establishment.

They persist to perpetuate arbitrary, inadequate, misleading and damaging concepts. There is absolutely no guarantee in today's world that we are receiving adequate amounts of these "non-essential nutrients" which in reality are essential. The fact is that we are *not* receiving them in significant quantities. The current *Plague of degenerative disease* is firm confirmation of this.

Due to the severe lack of phytonutrients, including plant derived minerals, vitamins, and other co-factors, all present for millions of years but now no longer significantly present in our food supply, we may not be able to adequately synthesize the other substances that are no less essential to health but which have been deceptively termed *"non-essential."*

An example of this is the termed *"non-essential"* amino acid proline, which is required for the synthesis of collagen. Without adequate amounts of proline and vitamin C, the production of collagen from pro-collagen is inhibited. Proline, lysine, green tea extract, and vitamin C inhibited the spread of cancer cells in an experimental study.

A much more realistic and less misleading definition for the term *"essential nutrient"* would be; *any and all nutrients required by the human cell and thus the human body, to perform any and all vital physiologic functions.* Herein lies the problem for *The Cartel;* defined in this manner, an emphasis of importance and criticality becomes apparent to the public, and the focus and reliance upon profitable drugs as *"the solution"* diminishes.

The term *"non-essential nutrient"* is one that, in reality, has little or no relevance in today's nutrient-poor society. All nutrients required by the human cell are essential, and we can no longer afford to rely on the body to synthesize nutrients where co-factor components may no longer exist. In addition, who within the medical or scientific community could pretend to understand the functional roles of all of the many hundreds, if not thousands, of phytonutrients and co-factors (known and unknown) and just what classification of *"importance"* they should be assigned?

Another dangerous and misleading term is *"semi-essential."* For example, there are four amino acids considered to be "semi-essential" for children because the metabolic pathways that synthesize these amino acids are not *fully* developed. Woe to the child that is missing or deficient in one or more of these "semi-essential amino acids!" Since there is no guarantee that any child is receiving adequate levels of these in their diet, and they are *not* producing them themselves, these amino acids for children are not *"semi-essential,"* but quite certainly essential! Missing nutrients during childhood development potentially provide an open door for the manifestation of diseases in childhood, and the later appearance in adulthood. It is all economics. If big business can spare the expense of adding these four amino acids to an infant's formula, the industry cost savings are significant. The term *semi-essential* should be eliminated as well in regard to nutrients.

There are two *"officially recognized"* essential fatty acids; alpha linolenic (Omega III) and linolenic (Omega VI). Under optimum conditions your body can manufacture the other fatty acids required for health if you have adequate amounts present of these two essential fatty acids. It has been estimated that an optimum ratio of dietary Omega III to Omega VI fatty acids would not exceed 1:3. The reality is that most Americans consume a dietary ratio estimated to be 1:20! We are falling considerably short on Omega III. Furthermore, due to the nutrient and trace nutrient poor diet that is consumed by most, it is highly likely that the conversion of the inadequate levels of essential fatty acids will not likely be converted to the other necessary fatty acids, and therefore we are deficient in them as well!

We would all prefer optimum health and a disease-free existence. As we can now see clearly, what others consider *"non-essential"* for us is Not what we would consider non-essential *for ourselves.* Merely relying upon the *"officially recognized"* essentials, may be engineered survival, but not engineered quality of life. Interestingly, this *surviving but suffering* public certainly creates an endless demand for expensive pharmaceuticals and medical procedures.

In simple terms;

1. **Perfect nutritional cellular support prevents and can eliminate most disease and premature aging ...**

2. **Perfect nutritional cellular support progressively minimizes or prevents the need for expensive drugs and invasive surgical procedures ...**

3. <u>**Prevention**</u> **eliminates the need for the bulk of pharmaceuticals.**

Would Big Pharma like to hinder or even *eliminate* Prevention?

This question is left open for *you.*

How did the term *"side effects"* come about?

Should we attend a magic show at the local fair, a magician may entertain us with illusions. Illusions are tricks designed to cause us to believe something is, or has occurred, that in reality is not or has not. The basis of a good trick or illusion is to distract the viewer while the reality of the situation goes unnoticed. Humans are designed with two eyes situated in the front of their skulls. We look forward when we think and focus. We usually focus on what is being presented directly in front of us. We are easily distracted, sometimes with the use of props. We cannot focus clearly on any subject using our peripheral vision. When something is off to the side and not emphasized, we tend to miss it. Things we miss or do not see clearly, we cannot focus on. Sometimes, things we do not see, we may not believe *really* exist.

Back in the day when the aspiring *masters* of illusion, the pharmaceutical marketers, first realized their products carried harmful and sometimes lethal effects, they were presented with a daunting dilemma. As they do today, they desired desperately to peddle their synthetic concoctions in the largest possible volume, regardless of consequence to the public. Their self-serving, profit-driven desire was to minimize the focus on the harmful properties within their synthetic products. Certainly, they must have initially wished they could just push these marketing dilemmas off the table, or at least, off to *the side*. Resorting to psychology, they soon discovered that inference is often a master of problem solving. They realized if they would just infer or imply that these harmful effects are *"really not a big deal"* by simply labeling them as <u>side</u> effects, then, the public would perceive them as *insignificant* and not what would be *truly expected* of the drug. The power of suggestion! Brilliant!! - Yet in this case, completely uninspiring. Once again, in reality, *"side effects"* are the direct unwanted effects of the drug.

Pay no attention to the man behind the curtain!

Today, when most people hear the term *side effects,* their perception and hope is that the drug will have a good chance to *"work,"* or even *"get a running start"* before the side effects have a chance to show up, *heck-* if they will even show up at all! The stark reality is; the biological monkey wrench is causing damage to the pristine cellular machine from the moment we swallow the synthetic substance. The mere hope of the drug *"working"* is a *Grand Illusion* in itself as well. Ninety-nine percent of all drugs marketed only mask (cover-up) symptoms of underlying problems. They do not *"work"* at all (see Chapter 5, The Current State of Modern Medicine).

These are *The Masters of Distraction.* Diverting public attention away from the reality of prevention and healing is the crux of their illusion. Obviously, prevention and healing should be intelligently addressed through cellular support by the natural means for which we are designed.

While modern symptom relief may have its temporary place to help us cope while suffering pain, dysfunction from illness, or injury; symptom relief should not be the mainstay of *"disease care"* which it has forcefully become. Common sense confirms this, yet this is the current portrait of *"healthcare,"* painted by these illusionists. Apparently, we are not supposed to be paying close attention.

Ironically, the vast majority of medications treat only symptoms and possess no curative powers. If a person heals at all, it is due to time and the body's innate healing processes. This is one important fact the pharmaceutical industry does not want emphasized; namely that given the proper natural resources, barring overwhelming trauma, intoxification or infection, the body *can and will* heal itself!

Symptom Relief Roulette (SRR)

I refer to the "drug-insanity" to which the modern-day medical patient falls victim as Symptom Relief Roulette. History has shown that the drugs *"approved"* by the FDA (The Food and Drug Administration) are in many cases, no safer than those made in the basements and garages of less than ideal citizens, and often render lethal and damaging effects far greater. Many volumes could be written on this subject and the financial conflicts of interest existing within a bureaucracy intended to *protect* the public.

The result of decades of manufactured public blind faith in this *approval* system, in addition to the blind faith in practitioners who have forcibly become little more than Cartel salespersons, has rendered the masses perfect clients of Mr. Big. Remember Mr. Big? He was the villain in the movie "Live and Let Die," who was clever enough to make his drugs easily obtainable until his customers just could not cope without them. Then he dramatically raised the price!

The *Live and Let Die* mentality of *The Cartel* has such confidence in the public's blind faith, that they feel more than comfortable marketing the ridiculous. The television ads at present are no less than hilarious. Currently, they are telling us to take a pill rather than be annoyed with the prospect of having to urinate between baseball innings. If you feel a tingling in your legs, it is not because your body is telling you a circulation problem may exist and that you need to get more exercise, oh no, you presumably have *"restless leg syndrome,"* and your only salvation also lies in a pill. Unfortunately, this pill may at the very least induce uncontrollable gambling urges, in conjunction with extremely vivid, horrifically violent and brutal nightmares (all documented *side-effects*). If you suffer from osteoporosis (low bone mineral density), do not concern yourself with calcium and mineral supplementation - certainly not. Just pop the latest synthetic masterpiece, linked to osteonecrosis of the jaw, causing bone tissue to die and never regenerate and be done with it! If you would like to quit smoking, never mind will-power, your flavor-of-the-month awaits in a *doosie* that is likely, *according to their winking tortoise,* to send you into fits of chronic vomiting. Take all five together and you could sit in your chair for hours, feeling no tingles, passing no fluids, unable to rise, unable to speak, and vomiting on yourself in the name of modern medicine. Your bookie screaming over the cell phone has the best advice of all; *"Whatever you do, don't fall asleep!"*

Possibly they could all come up with a pill to take care of the *"rare but serious side effect"* they don not seem to want to talk about. Maybe it is among those that do not reveal themselves right away. Could it be one of those the FDA does not require announcing to the *silly unassuming consumer?*

Losing this dangerous game of health roulette is not always immediately apparent. Many times, the cellular damage caused by these synthetic concoctions may not surface for months or even years. When the damage does inevitably surface, you can be wholly certain that the traditional medical community will blame it on genetics *("your great grand-pop")*, your life style, or they may just shrug their shoulders and tell you; *"We really cannot determine, with any degree of certainty, what has caused your illness, but fortunately we have an entire slew of wonderful new drugs we can try out, and see what happens."*

In most cases you will simply never know what the *"side effects"* have done to your health, but you can be certain of one thing; no one producing any drug will voluntarily step forward and take responsibility. The "casino" *won't* be "comping" your room.

Again, much of the "need" for Symptom Relief Roulette could easily be avoided. Our *health care* system, if properly restructured, would profit enormously not by being a self-preserving drain on the patient, but by providing true heath care with the main focus on prevention.

The Tricks of the Trade

Most published *"controversy"* in regard to vitamins, minerals, and nutrients disseminates directly or indirectly from the Pharma/Medical Establishment or the marketing departments of various firms attempting to cast apprehension on competing products. How do they frighten us away from what is good for us – what was designed for us, and lure us towards harmful synthetic products-for-profit?

The key tool used is *misinformation*. For example, they will simply publish an article about "aluminum" without defining whether they are speaking about the organic or inorganic form. The public hears, "aluminum is bad" and they avoid products containing both organic and inorganic aluminum. The more they can make nature look *"potentially harmful,"* the better their toxin laden pharmaceuticals appear. The tactics are profitable and the result over time on public perception, and consequently public health, is a manufactured disaster.

Organic aluminum is present in many common fruits and vegetables such as bananas, cucumbers, and tomatoes. *Inorganic* aluminum is a toxic and potentially harmful metal. The plant has processed the inorganic mineral because we need the organic mineral. You cannot die eating organically grown bananas, cucumbers, and tomatoes. You can only become healthier!

Another classic example is the attack on natural Vitamin E and other naturally derived vitamins. In organic chemistry there are substances known as *"stereoisomers."* Basically, there may be two different forms of a substance (natural and synthetic) which may have the same number and types of atoms, but whose atomic arrangements in space are different.

There were misguided *"experiments"* conducted, using only an isolated version of *synthetically produced* vitamin E (a mixture of DL-alpha tochopherol acetate) in high amounts. None of the other seven naturally occurring components of vitamin E were added. The experiments were conducted using a synthetic vitamin E, therefore, any possible adverse reactions from these experiments are worthless and expected, because in nature, the other seven components in the E "complex" would be present. The *"adverse reactions"* were highly publicized by the mainstream medical community. They conveniently failed to inform the public that they were using synthetically produced vitamin E. They made nature look *"potentially harmful"* to the unsuspecting public - **Mission accomplished!** They did not go as far as to warn against almonds, avocado, olives, and spinach - all wonderful sources of natural Vitamin E. These types of covert and diabolical side-shows are a flagrant abuse of the public trust and inevitably culminate in the deterioration of public health.

Another published *"study"* was carried out using dehydrated eggs which inevitably showed an increase in cholesterol levels after consumption. Nowhere was it mentioned that dehydrated powdered eggs contain *oxidized* cholesterol, which was the cause of the elevation in abnormal lipids. Thus, "eggs" were labeled as the culprits for raising cholesterol levels. Who would eat rotten eggs containing rancid fat, except unsuspecting pawns in a misguided experiment designed to perpetuate misinformation to confuse and frighten the public? Typically, eggs do not raise cholesterol levels. They are a wonderful source of protein and other beneficial nutrients.

Tricks and misinformation in published *"health articles,"* which appear to be written by unbiased and reputable authors backed by big business interests often misdirect us from what is good. They are indirectly one of the leading causes of the rising rates of degenerative diseases.

"The Third World War is a global misinformation war lead by the multi-billion dollar pharmaceutical investment business with disease against all mankind." Dr. Matthias Rath.

Introduction

An Argument in the Industry

The wonderful and positive news which we are about to share with you can and will change your life. In all probability it will also extend your life if you take it to heart and take simple action. Unfortunately, before the reader can benefit from the positive, to a significant degree, he or she must understand the dark side of the current *"healthcare"* system.

According to the U.S. DEPARTMENT OF HEALTH AND HUMAN SERVICES, Centers for Disease Control and Prevention, National Center for Health Statistics; In 2017 Heart Disease, Cancer and Stroke are the #1, #2, and #5 leading causes of death in the United States.

In an article in ***The Journal of the American Medical Association*** (JAMA), Dr. Barbara Starfield of the Johns Hopkins School of Hygiene and Public Health reported up to 225,000 deaths per year in the U.S. from *iatrogenic causes,* which rank these deaths as the #3 killer. (Iatrogenic death is a term defining patient death as a direct result of treatments by a physician, whether from misdiagnosis of the ailment, or adverse drug reactions used to treat the illness. Drug reactions are the most common cause of iatrogenic death).

Although an argument seems to exist as to who rightfully receives credit for the *show* position, (#3), concerning hundreds of thousands of needless deaths, the diseases or the doctors, one thing is curious for certain: As of the printing of this publication, the public is unable to access this information on the American Medical Association web-site. It is labeled, "Restricted."

Many familiar with this subject insist that the Pharma/ Medical establishment is the Number One (#1) cause of death due to their failure to inform the patient about the truths of health. For this reason, they argue, The Establishment is responsible, directly or indirectly, for every death involving disease which may have been prevented or cured, had the patient been properly informed. They base their argument for this responsibility on The Establishment's dissemination of misinformation about true health, which is a direct violation of the doctor-patient relationship based on trust. Most doctors are not aware of, or perpetrating any conspiracy. They are simply being misled.

As you read the information to follow, it may become more than apparent that if the American Medical Association (AMA) would allow doctors to PROPERLY instruct patients in regard to health, over time we would see no diseases outranking accidents, drastic reductions in all disease figures across the board, and very little deaths caused by doctors.

To give credit where credit is due, probably the greatest technological advance in modern medicine is the treatment for crisis situations. Surgical procedures have been developed that accomplish miraculous results. Where would we be, for example, without the skilled emergency room doctor, surgeon, and staff when we are burned, poisoned, injured by accident, or devastated by a virus such as COVID-19? Emergency care and/or surgery can be life saving in the case of accident, heart attack, stroke, or the removal of a tumor to name just a few.

Unfortunately, we have been conditioned to rely on drugs and surgery to correct the majority of our ills. The need for most surgeries could certainly be avoided in the first place if the patient were not permitted to deteriorate for decades due to misinformation and a complete lack of prevention.

"The doctor of the future will give no medicine but will interest his patient in the human frame, in diet and the cause and prevention of disease." Thomas Edison

"Let your food be your medicine, and your medicine be your food." Hippocrates – "The Father of Medicine."

Most doctors practicing today, regardless of their specific field, are wonderful caring individuals. It is the entrenched profit-based policies of The Establishment system which are to blame for the miserable track record of modern medicine ... <u>not</u> the doctors.

Robert E. Wilner, M.D., Ph.D. stated; *"Physicians today are required to practice within the "standards of the community." This does not mean what it seems to say. The word standard no longer refers to the qualities of high or low, excellent or poor. It now means that you do what everybody else is doing; even though no vote on the matter has been taken . . . The physician of today is merely the product of over a century of conditioning in "legitimate drug" culture. The neuroses of arrogance and dogma have made medicine self-destructive and severely impaired its capacity for creative or dissident thinking. It has always been the dissident thinker which has caused the art and the science of medicine to advance and flourish."*

"It is historical fact that the pharmaceutical industry (the oil and chemical industry) has been the major force responsible for the narrow, arrogant and simple minded path that has brought physicians success in less than ten percent of the diseases they are called upon to treat. The pharmaceutical complex provides research grants, contracts and advertising support responsible for the existence for the many thousands of journals published each year. This guarantees virtual control over scientific and medical direction and thought. The result has been highly profitable. By creating a dogmatic religious zeal in the search for the "holy grail," the cure of all disease by drugs, the average physician has become totally intolerant of all other schools of thought and practice. The great majority of physicians are honest, dedicated, and sincere scientists. They truly believe that they are on the "cutting edge" of medicine and that anyone who pursues another path is either misguided or ill- informed . . . as long as physicians pursue the magic bullet and ignore thousands of years of experience; iatrogenic (medically caused) illness and death will become more prevalent than ever."

Albert Einstein stated; *"To me the worst thing seems to be a school principally to work with methods of fear, force and artificial authority. Such treatment destroys the sound sentiments, the sincerity and the self-confidence of pupils and produces a subservient subject."*

Doctors today are working with the tools they are permitted to utilize by *establishment policy*, primarily drugs. The majority of these brilliant, well-intentioned practitioners have become the *subservient subjects.* This will be further discussed, but for now it is most important to understand the magnitude of the current epidemic of disease upon our society and most importantly, the solution.

Currently, one in three Americans are expected to contract some type of (cancer) in their lifetime. Cancer alone causes 22% of deaths. Prostate cancer eventually afflicts some 50-70% of men, while breast cancer attacks one out of every eight women. Over 100 million Americans suffer from some form of digestive disease, 80 million Americans suffer from arthritis, 61 million Americans (almost one-fourth of the adult population) live with active cardiovascular disease, 21 million suffer from diabetes, 18 million from obstructive sleep apnea (OSA), and 50 million Americans are afflicted with tinnitus, to mention the tip of the iceberg. The young are developing diseases which will be diagnosed in their later years.

Diseases are out of control in America and they are fueled by the allopathic philosophy of the main-stream medical establishment, which focuses on symptoms rather than prevention and the *causes* of disease. This philosophy is the imposed will of Big Pharma. More and more people do not have the energy they need to get through the day while millions of others are suffering with degenerative disease. Millions more await diagnosis due to the fact that the overwhelming majority of the population are experiencing cellular starvation and premature aging, - no matter how much food they consume. (See "Overeating Yet Under-Feeding," page 103).

In an effort to condense lengthy verbiage, we will henceforth be referring to this modern-day plague, as; ***The Plague of Degenerative Diseases,*** or simply, ***"The Plague"*** which also encompasses or represents the deteriorative forces of pre-mature aging.

Understanding the Cure

As previously defined; the term *phytonutrient* is derived from the Greek word *phyto* meaning plant, and *nutrient;* a constituent of food, vital for physiological function. Phytonutrients are biologically active compounds in plant-derived foods that elicit biological activity in the body.

Phytonutrients are necessary for optimum health due to their vast array of cellular functions. Phytonutrients stimulate our immune and natural detoxification systems. According to United States Department of Agriculture (USDA), phytonutrients may serve as antioxidants, enhance immune response, enhance cell to cell communication, cause cancer cells to die, and repair DNA damage. As we will be discussing, many of the benefits mentioned here are just the tip of the iceberg.

USDA, Quote: "While these **phytonutrients** aren't *"essential"* by traditional definitions, *they apparently* reduce risks of diseases of aging."

Now let us ponder that statement for a moment. With degenerative diseases escalating out of control in this country, with millions of lives lost and billions being ineffectually spent annually, we would be rather inclined to scrap the *"traditional definition"* and term them Essential. Of course, the focus of all this is mysteriously kept on the sidelines while we deteriorate, inspired to wait for Big Pharma to come up with another dandy, and the nauseating antics of Hollywood divas dominate *"the news."*

Did you catch the "down-play" in that last USDA sentence? It was the bolded words; *they apparently.* It is as if they are distressed in having to announce this. Hundreds, if not thousands of reputable scientific studies confirm it, and they are using the words *they apparently.* Well this is APPARENTLY very good news for a society of taxpayers suffering from pre-mature aging and a host of degenerative diseases. *Apparently,* it would have been a very good idea to send every citizen a notice in the mail! If they were worried about the postage costs, they could have coordinated with the IRS and slipped the notice in with the tax correspondence.

The USDA goes on to state that *isoflavones* may reduce the risk of heart disease, osteoporosis, and several types of cancer, and certain flavonoids in blueberries may actually reverse nerve cell aging and a wide array of compounds in fruits and vegetables may protect cell components against oxidative damage as well as vitamins C or E.

Yes, you read correctly. <u>Flavonoids reverse cell aging</u>. Keep in mind that all these wonderful benefits stated are isolated to only what they currently understand *or choose to disclose* concerning these majestic bio-active living constituents.

Upon reading this, an intelligent person may surmise that these are *just a few minor points* that make the difference between disease, suffering, and pre-mature death, versus a long and healthy life. Throughout this book we will periodically prompt you to ask yourself a question such as: **Why has this information been kept on the sidelines?**

The United States Department of Agriculture (USDA) Quote: *"Plant foods contain biologically active components beyond those defined as essential nutrients, such as thousands of anti-oxidant phytochemicals that impart health benefits <u>beyond the basic nutrition for an intended population.</u>"*

This is a very interesting statement for a government branch to publish because it indicates to the reader that the government has allowed to exist, or intended for the population, for whatever reason, a sub-essential (or incomplete) list of nutrient standards defined as the *"essential nutrients."*

They continue;

The United States Department of Agriculture (USDA) Quote: *"...there exists a large and growing body of evidence showing that the foods we choose each day play a critical role in disease prevention. Plant foods, again, contain "extra" bioactive substances that, while not on the government's list of essential nutrients, may still be protective against cancer risk.* ***These disease fighting nutrients can boost our antioxidant activity, immune systems, elimination of toxic substances, and inhibition of tumor cells and carcinogentic fat.***"

This statement, in conjunction with the previous, indicates to the reader that *The True Essential Nutrient List* designed by "The Supreme Intelligence" or "nature," whichever you choose, to impart optimum health benefits is very long in comparison with the government's short-list disclosure.

They further state;

The United States Department of Agriculture (USDA) Quote: *"Population studies have linked fruit and vegetable consumption with lowering the risk for chronic diseases including specific cancers and heart disease." ..."For now, it appears that an effective strategy for reducing the risk of cancer and heart disease is to increase consumption of phytonutrient-rich foods including fruits vegetables, grains, and teas."*

The Centers for Disease Control and Prevention; Quote: *"Current evidence collectively demonstrates that fruit and vegetable intake is associated with improved health, reduced risk of major diseases, and possibly delayed onset of age-related factors."*

As *mildly indicated* here by these two government bodies, and confirmed by hundreds of research studies conducted worldwide, **the cures are clearly designed into the plants** and subsequently the foods, in the form of these disease fighting bioactive substances. Provided that the necessary minerals and nutrients are found in the soil, the vital phytonutrients will be produced in the plant, *but again, herein lyes the problem.*

The food we eat today is far removed from what our grandparents or great-grandparents ate. In those days, all food was organically grown. There were no artificial fertilizers, pesticides, herbicides, hormones, antibiotics, or genetically modified food crops. Most food was grown locally and was consumed within a few days of being picked or caught. It was not sprayed with preservatives, mold inhibitors or waxes. The soil was rich with nutrients and essential minerals yielding crops high in the same. The healthy soil had a living environment containing nitrogen-fixing bacteria, minerals, and was alive with rich organic matter. This is no longer the case. The overwhelming majority of the modern day food supply is grown in depleted soils void of the necessary components needed to produce sufficient vital life-saving phytonutrients.

Should we still be wondering why pre-mature aging and degenerative diseases are spiraling out of control? All this while the Pharma/Medical establishment is pretending to be *"in search of the cures"* and our doctors are sending us home with more and more prescriptions for toxic drugs which address no causes and cure virtually nothing.

The prevention of, and the cure for the majority of degenerative diseases and conditions alike, **is already known.** For the main part due to the synergistic effect that these disease fighting bioactive living substances possess when combined, **the prevention or cure is basically the same for most.**

The cure, and preferably the prevention of the majority of degenerative diseases and conditions, is the consistent daily ingestion of a comprehensive, full spectrum of disease fighting plant-derived bioactive substances, in sufficient amounts, while avoiding harmful substances both on the market and in most cases, those approved by the FDA. (See "The Slow Death List" page 107).

We refer to this full spectrum of age and disease fighting bioactive substances as *"The Universal Spectrum of Life."* It is this natural and powerful *Spectrum of healing phytonutrients* that the Pharma/Medical establishment is attempting to minimize from publication and thus public awareness, for it is this wonderful Spectrum which renders their *"magic-bullet,* one-patent-for-profit-synthetic-toxic-laden-drug-for-each-pain-and-symptom-philosophy,"* **USELESS.** It is the very existence of this natural and powerful Spectrum of Healing, so well understood by the scientific community, which exposes the farce of *"the search for the cures,"* in which the drug industry portrays their image. (More on *"The Universal Spectrum of Life"* to follow).

You live in the age of the KNOWN CURES

Many cures have been known by scientists and doctors who have been threatened with research funds being cut-off, jobs terminated, and licenses to practice revoked. Today, many a good practicing physician would love nothing more than to be granted permission to treat their patients effectively. Many a good man and women who have attempted to go against the Pharma/Medical Establishment and bring true healing and prevention to the deficient, sick, and suffering public, have suffered the consequences themselves and have been ostracized. These are *"The Martyrs of Modern Medicine,"* and when the head has finally been removed from this giant parasitic beast on public health, through exposure, these souls will be vindicated and the public freed.

"We are asking the public to believe in what we do not believe in ourselves. We are asking them to take medicines we will ourselves will not take and to submit to operations which we will not permit on ourselves." E. G. Jones, M.D.

"Every degenerative disease can be traced back to an organic mineral deficiency." Two-time Nobel Prize winner, Linus Pauling

Who's in Charge?

Imagine living in a prison environment in a foreign country where you receive your news and information from one source. Your television has only one channel and the prison staff, in particular the warden, controls everything you view. If the warden docs not want the prison population to view a particular telecast, it will not be broadcast on The Channel. If the warden did not want a particular piece of information to be known, he would sensor that as well. Picture yourself as an inmate in the prison population (relax, we know you're innocent). You would not know if the information you were viewing was accurate, incomplete, or altogether false. If the news looked real on The Channel you may not even suspect that it was false, incomplete or slanted in any manner. What the warden decided to broadcast would be all the information you would ever receive. Life would go by while the entire inmate population was misled and "kept in the dark."

Sounds like a horrible situation to be in, does it not?

Americans receive their news from several main sources; Television, Radio, Newspaper, and Internet newspaper/network sites.

It will be no shock to anyone to learn that one of the top purchasers of advertising medium in all the media sources listed above is Big Pharma. One of the richest industries in the world, the pharmaceutical industry commands a top position in advertising dollars spent and subsequently, "top clout". They certainly do want us to receive their message. (Equally as important to them, are messages which they do not want us to receive). This means that they are a very important client of the media in general. News stations owned by networks as well as independent stations both rely on advertising dollars to survive. It is the same with print and other forms of media as well. It is simply how they make their money. The more viewers or readers the media source receives, the higher their *"ratings"* or *"readership"* figures, and thus the more money they are able to command for their advertising time or space. Consequently, a *"news station," "news broadcast,"* or *"news publication"* is a business for profit. Hence, the *"news"* we view, depending on the topic, may not be the real news at all. For the most part we view what has been approved to be released for us to view. It is *"The Golden Rule"* of the money world which applies - *He who has the gold - Makes the Rules.*

Few have more gold than Big Pharma. Metaphorically, this places Big Pharma in the position of *"The Warden."* No business wants to lose their biggest client. No business wants to lose one of their largest sources of advertising dollars, especially when the competing media is raking in those Pharma dollars. Currently, the national media is *addicted* to the advertising dollars of pharmaceutical companies. The networks and independents alike are heavily dependent upon drug advertising. In most cases, upon review, findings or information contrary to the drug agenda will simply be left out or buried, rather than risk the potential upset of the big client. Henceforth in many cases, as with any other industry, the mere presence of money and power influences action or inaction. Income represents the quality of content a media outlet can produce. If they cannot match the competition in desirable content, viewer ratings will drop and in time, they are out of the game. This gives Big Pharma, *Big Clout,* placing the drug industry in the position of unwritten censorship control. They are largely, The Warden of what we view regarding health.

The Cartel holds the cards. They have the power to influence what is printed, broadcast, and what remains unseen. Should that tainted information we believe to be *"the news"* or the lack of vital information withheld from us cause a lifetime of pain, deterioration, or premature death, *then so be it* seems to be the drug industry attitude. Profits from drug sales are King. This is their system. We can be wise or blind to these facts - the choice is ours. This is the state of the world we live in. The harsh reality is the world and what we see is controlled by money and greed, not compassion, and thus the **The Plague** proliferates.

Oh, those beautifully choreographed, softly lit, just out-of-focus Big Pharma ads. Who else is capable of such masterful displays of heartfelt emotion? Who else has an unlimited production and advertising budget? Oh the way they *feel and flow*, with just the right touch of slow-mo. The happy, healthy participants portray the vision of *the way a splendid life should be.* "Now *Keepemsic®"may not be for everyone,* so ask your doctor if *Keepemsic®* is right for you!"

Since your doctor may be receiving significant compensation in the form of perks (an estimated 20 billion annually) for prescribing *Keepemsic®*, chances are it may be just what the doctor orders, and if you are extra lucky, you may even leave his office with an additional prescription for *Killemoff®*.

Did you know they are telling us *the truth* when they say *"may not be for everyone?"* The fact that this clever statement is *less than a half-truth* really does not seem to matter. The whole truth is; side-effect-laden synthetic chemicals *"are not for"* ANYONE. They are against the human design and thus produce one hundred thousand plus annual deaths, and approximately 2.2 million annual hospitalizations involving adverse reactions. Some say the number of unreported deaths and maiming is incalculable. We would say, to a good degree, the bodily maiming figure is *entirely* calculable; if one hundred million Americans are on some form of side-effect-laden synthetic chemical, then one hundred million Americans are receiving some degree of cellular damage and/or disruption as a direct effect of the against-the-design substance.

Did you know that in recent years the Pharma Cartel has been charged with registered complaints of crimes against humanity for systematically obstructing and even fighting the prevention and the eradication of diseases?

Big Pharma invests millions in campaign contributions designed to benefit their interests and promote their agendas. Not only will some candidates promise to support certain policies and bills prior to being elected, but after gaining office they will then be obligated to repay the favors in the form of passing various legislations which benefit their big contributor and hinder natural practitioners and manufacturers.

The corruption does not stop with politicians. In a 2006 article printed in the Boston Globe entitled, *"How Drug Lobbyists Influence Doctors,"* it was estimated that the pharmaceutical companies spend nearly 20 billion dollars annually to influence the nation's 600,000 to 700,000 physicians to prescribe the newest and most expensive drugs.

These corrupt systems of influence are outrageous conflicts-of-interest literally killing the American public. The annual bill for treating medication misuse is a stunning $177 billion. We are deteriorating and dying while being misled, robbed, and taken for fools. The latest variety of drug propaganda ads utilize cartoons in an attempt to appeal to a paying public whom they perceive as mindless. *"Ask your doctor if XYZ drug is right for you."*

"...the forces of the drug cartel that - through its influences in world media – has launched a mis-information campaign of unprecedented proportions to discredit the scientific truth and attack those who have become pioneers in spreading this breakthrough." Dr. Matthias Rath.

Thousands of scientists, researchers, and even the USDA have conceded that phytonutrients enhance cell-to-cell communication and immune response, detoxify carcinogens, repair DNA damage, and cause cancer cells to die. This, the tip of the iceberg. Can you imagine if a synthetic drug were created which would accomplish just a fraction of all this? Why, it would be the largest selling pharmaceutical of all time, *despite* the inevitable side effects.

The good news is that there is no need to wait for Big Pharma's next Deadly Blunder. Nature's potent, healing cellular-spectrum of phytonutrient life has already been created!

A Note to the Reader

In the later stages of writing this book, I took notice of a wonderful publication written by author, Rhonda Byrne, entitled "The Secret." Ms. Byrne's book addresses the powers of positive thought and how the "laws of attraction" govern our universe. We really liked everything about the book.

In her book, Ms. Byrne describes "a secret" that great minds of the past and present have all known in regard to powers, which have been largely hidden from the world society by "the powers that be" (The Establishments) in all periods. I found the similarity fascinating as to how both our topics, unrelated in subject matter, were identical in regard to big business withholding life-empowering information from the public.

Jesus and Buddha, inventors such as Thomas Edison and Henry Ford, and scientists such as Albert Einstein, all seem to concur with the book's positive–thought conclusions. I personally know of two people whose emotional lives have been saved by the information in that little book, but that is not my point here.

My point is, I found it interesting to witness the most outspoken critics of her wonderful work were those who presumably represent establishment medicine; The *"medical professionals."* God Forbid the people should be enlightened and empowered in a positive way.

While reading a few of the published critical comments from a few psychologists, I could not help but suspect that their true fears lie in large, in the concern that the useful information contained within Rhonda Byrne's book might cause positive thought and action, and thus a loss of control and quite possibly a decline in their patient portfolios. Indeed, it is those who are in control in general, who do not want certain secrets revealed. Dr. Ronald Ducker

By providing the critical and timely health information contained within *The Code of Life...,* We too hope to enlighten and empower the people, particularly the sick and/or aging. (All of us).

A few of the co-authors of *the Secret* make it clear that positive thought is imperative but *"action will sometimes be required."* *"...when the intuitive nudge from within is there, act."*

It is my hope that this book, **The Code of Life...,** will be your "intuitive nudge from within" to take charge of your health!

Chapter 1

The Code,
The Spectrum, and
The Symphony of Life

"Look deep, deep into nature, and then you will understand everything better." Albert Einstein

Note: The terms and concepts in the following section are intended for the purpose of reader perspective and visualization.

We must first understand that which has been hidden from us;
The Keys to Health, Youth, and Longevity

"The Universal Spectrum of Life" represents the vast number of nutritional elements required by the human cell to perform all physiologic functions by design, avoid cellular starvation, thus deterioration, pre-mature aging, and disease. Adequate and quality cellular nutrition in relation to cell health, longevity, and disease prevention is a proven and undisputed scientific fact recognized for decades by the scientific community.

Within *The Universal Spectrum of Life* are specific or "special" phytonutrients including immune modulating components, which are designed to be used by the cells as components of communication. These components enable cells to communicate with other cells and with the immune system to perform an entire array of health functions including; the elimination of foreign invaders such as viruses, harmful bacteria, and diseased cells. These special components of communication metaphorically make up the "symbols" of this physiologic language. These are the symbols of *"The Code of Life,"* which represents the vast and complex

52

physiological science of cells communicating with other cells within our bodies. This fascinating discovery has become more fully studied and understood within the last decade. (See Chapter 6, The Amazing Immune System.)

Note: Upon regular ingestion of these stabilized components, we have witnessed patients dramatically improve, and in many cases, literally walk away from diseases altogether (digestive and autoimmune diseases in particular), nearly all of which the traditional medical community label as *"incurable"* such as; Inflammatory Bowel Disease (IBD: Crohn's Disease and Ulcerative Colitis), Irritable Bowel Syndrome (IBS), Gastroesophageal Reflux Disease (GERD), Heartburn, Diverticulitis, Chronic Fatigue Syndrome (CFS), Gastric Ulcers, Constipation, Diarrhea, Allergies, Food Intolerances, Lactose Intolerance, Malabsorption, Arthritis, Lupus, and every nearly every common and often times uncommon disease on the autoimmune list. (see list page **62**)

Numerous multi-functional nutritional components of *The Code of Life* also play an array of cellular support, detoxification, and nourishment roles within *The Universal Spectrum of Life,* as many of the components of *The Spectrum* equally help promote optimal communication within *The Code.*

Both working together in synergism orchestrate *"The Symphony of Life."* *The Symphony,* which represents the complete bio-chemical activity of the cell and its interaction with other cells, orchestrates every single physiologic function occurring within the human body. The healthy or *optimum orchestration* of *The Symphony of Life* within us is entirely dependent upon the quality and quantity of nutritional components (including *The Code*)within*The Universal Spectrum of Life.*

Illustrated:

The Code of Life
(Specific & often uncommon cellular
communication components (nutrients))

within:

The Universal Spectrum of Life
(The full spectrum of age and disease fighting
nutrients and bio-active phytonutrients)

Yields or Orchestrates:

The Symphony of Life
(The complete, harmonious, and synergistic bio-chemical
activity orchestrating every physiological function occurring
throughout the entire human body)

All are critical to our health and survival, and in essence,
All work together as One!

These are the basic concepts of health which
have been obscured by the pharmaceutical drug establishment.

They are factually the hidden keys to health, healing, disease
prevention, youth, beauty, anti-aging, and longevity.

Phytonutrients are necessary for optimum health due to their vast
array of cellular functions. This is what humans are designed to
receive. Therefore, phytonutrients are ESSENTIAL and necessary for
sustaining human life as well as combating pre-mature aging and
disease. They are the intended fuel and medicine by design.

A Synthetic *"Vitamin"* is not a Vitamin

Most *"food supplements"* sold on the market today are synthetic, which are much cheaper to produce than natural *plant-derived* (phytonutrients) vitamins or supplements.

You may be surprised to know that China is one of the largest exporters of many drugs and *"vitamins."* China's supplement industry suffers from the same type of conflict-of-interest that we endure with regard to the drug industry here in the United States where politicians and regulators have financial interests in the industries they are paid to "regulate and inspect." Much of the industry structure in China yields little if any reliable way for a consumer to determine from where a given product originated or from what it was produced.

If a scientist knows the chemical pathway, and he is not so much concerned *with what he does not understand or will inevitably create,* then it is possible for him to produce almost anything in an inexpensive, synthetic manner in a laboratory. One unnatural process utilized in regard to "vitamins" is known as *"mirror imaging."*

Through mirror imaging, synthetic vitamins and minerals are synthesized by the pharmaceutical and chemical industries from many of the same starting materials that drugs are made from, primarily; coal tar, petroleum products, animal by-products, waste, shells, and inorganic minerals.

Synthetic vitamins possess limited, laboratory created *mirror-image components* (isolated synthetic parts). They are wholesaled to the various nutrient manufacturers most of whom have no scientific knowledge of how or from what these various *"vitamins and minerals"* are made. Many just assume a vitamin is a vitamin. Many so-called *"natural"* vitamins have synthetics added to the blend, as they only need to be 10% natural by law to make the *"natural"* claim.

Conversely, most vitamins and nutrients found in nature's plants are found in complex groups or "families." The scientific identifications of these individual components within these families are comprised solely of those which are presently known. Those known are limited in number in contrast to the Grand Natural Design, for certainly there will be many more discoveries of additional components found within the entire plant complex.

Phytonutrients created by nature, including complex carbohydrates, amino acids, fatty acids, enzymes, antioxidants, vitamins, and minerals contain a total "complex" or family of micro-nutrient co-factors as they are found in nature. A prime example of this is Aloe vera. Aside from the polymannan molecule, there are some 200 other known ingredients which make up the synergistic "complex" known as *The Healing Orchestra* of Aloe.

Another example would be some of the co-factors found to accompany plant-derived Vitamin C, which are various bio-flavonoids. These micro-nutrient co-factors are indispensable for proper Vitamin C absorption and maximum utilization.

Synthetic vitamins are in most cases, *"orphans of function."* They lack these miraculous natural supporting families or complexes which are as recent science has demonstrated, the pathways to optimal health by design.

As stated, synthetic vitamins possess a laboratory created mirror-image component, out of an entire complex or family of micro-nutrients or co-factors that accompany the vitamin in its natural phytonutrient state.

Scientific research has shown that plant-derived natural vitamin complexes, with all co-factors present, are much more effective than high doses of synthetic and *"fractionated"* vitamins. (The term *fractionated* refers to an isolated portion or just a part of the original natural molecular complex).

By nature's hand, these perfectly designed *human-fuel*-phytonutrients possess high levels of *biological activity*, which is the measure of potency or functional use in the body. They are the *living* cellular fuel of rejuvenation.

"Synthetic vitamins may perform some of the functions of their natural counterparts while being useless for others. But what may be more important is the fact that synthetic vitamins, prepared from chemicals instead of nature, are frequently less active biologically than their natural counterparts, thereby reducing any beneficial effect they may have." British researcher Isobel Jennings, of Cambridge University.

For example, Vitamin E is a fat-soluble vitamin that exists in eight different forms. <u>Each form has its own biological activity</u>. Antioxidants such as vitamin E in their natural state act to protect your cells against the effects of free radicals, play a role in immune function, in DNA repair, and other metabolic processes.

The synthetic form of Vitamin E displays only one-third to one-half the biological activity as the natural form. The synthetic form is an isolated version of the natural, containing "a copy" of *only one* of the eight different forms of natural Vitamin E. Furthermore, the synthetic form interferes with the utilization of the natural one. Some health problems have been associated with the synthetic form.

The "experiments" (side shows in this case) in which harmful effects have been demonstrated with the use of *"vitamin supplementation,"* have used the *synthetic, isolated* form of the vitamin for the experiment. This is true of vitamins A, beta-carotene, C, D, and E. These experiments are representative of what occurs when man, in his efforts to create a cheaper-to-produce-substance, attempts to *"duplicate"* nature. These *"vitamin studies"* sponsored by the pharmaceutical industry often come to the conclusion that *"vitamins are not safe."* This is because they use *synthetic isolated "vitamins"* rather than whole natural sources. Purposely using the synthetic and isolated vitamins in these experiments paints a fraudulent picture of vitamins in general for the public. Although proven to be an effective scare tactic responsible for presumably many millions of lives lost, is it not sadly ironic that the pharmaceutical and chemical industries who are behind these fake *"experiments,"* are also the manufacturers of the compounds (or props in this case) which they are calling *"vitamins"* and publicly *"proving"* harmful? The small loss in vitamin revenue is re-captured many fold with increased pharmaceutical sales. They are hedged and positioned to profit either way.

The Body is a Whole

Under the heavy influence of Big Pharma, *the mainstream medical establishment* views the human body as more or less a machine-like mechanism made up of individual, and at times, replaceable parts. If an organ malfunctions, they administer a drug to alter its function, or if need be, remove it or attempt to replace it with a new organ. Although this restricted viewpoint of the human body is extremely self-limiting with regard to healing, it serves industry objectives well in the justification of expensive drugs and procedures as the main-stay *"solution."* Should the yoke of The Cartel ever be broken and *"modern medicine"* allowed to catch-up with science, (and common sense), these purposeful limitations will be discarded.

The human body is in fact much greater than simply the sum of its parts. We are vastly multi-dimensional, composed of matter and interacting energy. Our parts work in synergy, each cell, each organ dependent upon the welfare and health of the other. We are in part and in whole, a symphony of matter and energy, working, producing, communicating, and continually rendering that magnificent notion which we so casually define as "life." Our fuel and our medicine (natural) is life. Life has been created for life, and life sustains life.

> *"Each of us, a cell of awareness, imperfect and incomplete. Genetic blends, with uncertain ends, on a fortune hunt that's far too fleet."*
> Neil Peart

The Body is comprised of many systems, for example, the digestive, nervous, cardiovascular, respiratory, eliminatory, immune, cutaneous (skin), musculoskeletal, energy, or glandular systems. The optimal function of all these systems of the body are dependent upon and synergistic with one another, beginning with the digestive tract. The digestive tract must be operating at optimum health and efficiency in order to provide all areas of the body simultaneously with adequate nutrition.

Perfect Cellular Support

The degree to which our cells are effectively supported and communicating is the degree of protection we possess against aging and disease. Logically, anything less than 100% support and cellular communication is a partially opened door to pre-mature aging and disease. For this reason it would be preferable to consistently ingest *more* of the vital components than our bodies actually need, than to starve the cell to any degree. Scientific review supports the use of a wide variety of phytonutrients and it appears that the more antioxidant and phytonutrient protection we provide to our bodies, the better.

The perfect anti-aging, anti-disease philosophy becomes; ***"Every vital nutrient must be available within the body – for the support of the cell – All of the time."*** This implies any and all vital nutrients that the cell may require at any given time to perform any and all physiological functions must be present and available within the body at the moment of cellular demand. When the cell cries out for that one specific tool (nutrient) to perform its function and avoid deterioration, - that tool must be present.

Question: How do we prevent, fight against, and recover from disease? **Answer:**

1. First and foremost we take the necessary step to ensure that our digestive tracts are healthy and functioning at optimum, in order to absorb the vital nutrients from our foods and supplements. Immune modulating components are the foundation of this process.

2. We do our best to make certain that as many quality phytonutrients as reasonably possible are available within the body for the support of the cells. Nutrient starved cells deteriorate and die prematurely. Healthy eating and smart supplementation is the answer here. (to be covered)

Additionally, we must reduce or avoid the pitfalls of health to be discussed. (See "The Slow Death List" page 107.)

Healthy Digestion: The Masked Doorway to Health, Disease Prevention, and Recovery.

Ingestion of the very best foods and nutritional supplements may be rendered useless in large, without a healthy digestive environment. In order for these healing elements to be of benefit, we must be able to digest, absorb, and assimilate them into the bloodstream so that they may be incorporated into the approximate thirteen-trillion cells of our bodies.

Persons lacking healthy and efficient digestive function will progressively suffer the short and long-term effects of cellular starvation, premature aging and disease. In many instances, signs and symptoms of disease will manifest in the digestive tract itself as a direct result of the reduced ability to digest and process nutrients.

Some Very Good News

Healing made easy: Conversely, when we ingest concentrated natural immune modulating components, as an initial observation we progressively witness the reduction and eventual eradication of diseases of the digestive tract. Healthy digestion is the foundation of a healthy immune system and the first step in preventing and eliminating digestive, degenerative and autoimmune conditions. The consistent ingestion of the natural immune modulating components has proven to progressively accomplish both feats.

Our years of experience with the progressive elimination of symptoms and the subsequent eradication of "incurable" digestive, degenerative and autoimmune diseases have occurred with the utilization of a stabilized, concentrated formula of organic, natural immune modulating components known as "DigestaCure AUTOIMMUNE-X." The formula may be obtained without a prescription from LifeSavingFormulas.com in capsule or powder form.

We have patient-tested the initial prototypes of the formula developed over the last two decades, and have had the opportunity to provide input from our patient experiences during the numerous stages of formula development, and during current formula potency increase design.

In our practices, we have consistently proven this formula to be the answer to autoimmune diseases where there is no other medical remedy. The stabilized modulators exhibit no negative side-effects and have no contra-indications or reactions with medications or supplements. Occasionally a patient with bacterial build-up will report temporary, mild to moderate detoxification symptoms, but this can be fairly quickly overcome with temporary dosage reductions, additional hydration and if needed, activated charcoal capsules to absorb the released pathogen waste.

The formula is all-natural and outside the patentable control of the Pharmaceutical Industry thus the traditional medical doctor with drug-based training is generally unlikely to step outside the box and recommend it to patients. The formula is the enemy of The Cartel for it erodes the very *foundation* of their business with disease; *Autoimmunity.* That being said, there are currently over 600 natural practitioners and integrated medical doctors healing autoimmune conditions with the formula.

Using an organic, cultured 20th generation aloe botanical as source material, the nutraceutical manufacturer has effectively developed a processing method which stabilizes, preserves and concentrates the high molecular weight immune modulating components (one million to over ten million Dalton in molecular weight) and other essential healing components essential for the restoration of normal immune function, disease prevention, and recovery.

Should the reader enter the healing process with the immune modulators, please be certain to share your healing story with us. The details of your story will add to our knowledge and ability to share details with others with similar cases. Your report will also help us to keep average healing time-frame projections accurate for those just beginning the process with specific illnesses.

By eliminating the root-disease (the autoimmune attack on the tissues, systems, and organs of the body) we eliminate hundreds of symptoms and conditions, and place the body in a position to avoid every autoimmune disease on the list of over 100 as we age.

Below are the average healing time-frames reported for The Most Common Autoimmune Conditions.

If you do not see your condition listed here, see the entire list here; www.drronpdrucker.com/list or the symptoms list after.

Note: Those suffering with multiple autoimmune conditions generally heal from their conditions simultaneously, with some conditions ahead of others, case dependent. It is generally the conditions evolving tissues damage from the years of autoimmune attack which heal last, taking longer to heal in general.

Using the Immune Modulating Components The average healing time frames reported for The Most Common Autoimmune Conditions are:

Users with **Acid Reflux (GERD)** report an average healing time frame of 3 months to 100%.

Users with **Alopecia** (all types except male pattern baldness) report an average healing time of 12 months. Dormant hair follicles are reported to respond in widely varying time frames. Dead hair follicles as experienced with male pattern baldness, and to slight degrees with the other types of alopecia, will not be restored.

Users with **Amyotrophic Lateral Sclerosis** (Lou Gehrig's Disease) report widely varying healing time frames (dependent upon severity and degree of nerve damage) ranging from 40% to 70% improvement within 1 year. Improvements may continue slowly beyond 12 months.

Users with **Arthritis** (All types except Rheumatoid, see Rheumatoid below) report an average healing time of 8 months.

Users with **Asthma** report an average healing time frame of 10 months.

Users with **Autoimmune Hepatitis** report an average healing time frame of 12 months to a 75% recovery. Improvements may continue slowly beyond 12 months.

Users with **Barrett's esophagus** report an average healing time frame of 8 months. Varying levels of scar tissue may remain.

Users with **Bursitis** report an average healing time frame of 8 months.

Users with **Bullous Pemphigoid** report an average healing time frame of 8 months. The skin returns to normal.

Users with **Chronic Fatigue Syndrome and/or Fibromyalgia** report an average healing time of 8 months.

Users with **Celiac Disease** report an average healing time frame of 10 months. Varying levels of scar tissue may remain.

Users with **Colitis** (all types) report an average healing time frame of 5 months.

Users with **Crohn's Disease** report an average healing time frame of 5 months.

Users with **Cystitis** report an average healing time frame of 8 months.

Users with **Dermatitis, Eczema, and/or Psoriasis** report an average healing time frame of 8 months.

Users with **Diabetes Type 2** report an average healing time of 12 months with average improvements of 70-100% in blood sugar levels.

Users with **Diabetes Type 1** report an average healing time frame of 2 years with a 50-100% improvement in blood sugar levels. Varying levels of tissue damage may remain.

Users with **Diverticulitis** report an average healing time frame of 5 months.

Users with **Diverticulosis** report an average healing time frame of 3 months. Additional pouch formation halts and the existing diverticulum pouches progressively deinflame and subsequently strengthen but remain.

Users with **Fibromyalgia** report an average healing time frame of 8 months.

Users with **Gastritis** report an average healing time of 5 months.

Users with **General Digestive Dysfunction** report an average healing time frame of 3 months.

Users with **GERD (Gastro Esophageal Reflux Disease)** report an average healing time of 3 months.

Users with **Gout** report an average healing time of 8 months.

Users with **Graves' Disease** report an average healing time of 8 months.

Users with **Hashimoto's thyroiditis** report an average healing time frame of 8 months.

Users with **Hepatitis** report an average healing time of 12 months.

Users with **Hiatal Hernia** report an average healing time of 6 months for symptoms to subside. Varying levels of tissue damage may remain. The use of chiropractic adjustment to reposition the hernia back into the middle body cavity is advisable after inflammation has subsided.

Users with **High Blood Pressure (Hypertension)** report and average healing time frame of 8 months for blood pressure to normalize without the continued use of medications. Users report progressively weaning from blood pressure medications until no longer needed.

Users with **High Blood Cholesterol (LDL)** report and average healing time frame of 8 months for cholesterol levels to normalize without the continued use of medications. Users report progressively weaning from cholesterol medications until no longer needed.

Users with **Interstitial Cystitis** report an average healing time of 8 months.

Users with **Irritable Bowel Syndrome (IBS)** report an average healing time of 4 months.

Users with **Leaky-Gut Syndrome** report an average healing time frame of 4 months.

Users with **Lupus** report an average healing time of 5 months.

Users with **Lyme Disease** report widely varying healing time frames ranging from 4 months to 24 months with recovery levels ranging from 70% to 100%.

Users with **Multiple Sclerosis** report widely varying healing time frames (dependent upon severity and degree of nerve damage) ranging from 50% to 80% improvement within 1 year. Improvements may continue to improve slowly beyond 12 months.

Users with **Myasthenia Gravis** report an average healing time frame of 8 months. Eyelids are reported to return 80 to 100% normal position.

Users with **Nephritis** (with varying losses of kidney function) report healing time frames of 8 months to 18 months, with improvements in kidney function ranging from 50 to 100%.

Users with **Osteoporosis** report a cessation of bone loss or density in an average of 6 months, and significant increases in bone density in an average of 24 months.

Users with **Pernicious Anemia** report an average healing time frame of 8 months.

Users with **Proctitis** report an average healing time of 5 months.

Users with **Psoriasis** report an average healing time frame of 8 months.

Users with **Raynaud's Phenomenon** report an average healing time of 8 months. Improvements ranging from significant to full recovery in average healing time frames of 8 months. Varying levels of tissue damage can remain.

Users with **Rheumatoid Arthritis** report widely varying healing time frames (dependent upon severity and degree of joint damage) ranging from 30% to 90% improvement within 1 year. Improvements may continue slowly beyond 12 months. Varying levels of tissue damage may remain.

Users with **Rosacea** report an average healing time frame of 6 months.

Users with **Sarcoidosis** report an average healing time of 12 months. Varying levels of lung tissue damage may remain.

Users with **Scleroderma** report a cessation in the hardening affect in an average time frame of 6 months. Tissue softening is reported to be a very long process and varying levels of tissue damage will remain.

Users with **Sjogren's Syndrome** report an average healing time of 8 months.

Users with **Ulcerative Colitis** and **Crohn's Disease** report an average healing time frame of 5 months.

Users with **Vasculitis** report an average healing time of 6 months.

Users with **Vitiligo** report an average healing time frame of 4 months for cessation of the spreading. Progressive improvements in pigment levels are reported as the months progress, provided small intervals of sun exposure are obtained. No one to date has reported the return of pigment in excess of a 70% degree in the effected areas.

Users with **Yeast Overgrowth,** leaky gut and food intolerances report an average healing time frame of 5 months.

If you do not have an official diagnosis, find your symptoms on the autoimmune symptoms list on the next page:

Common Autoimmune Symptoms List:

abdominal cramping
abdominal pain
abdominal swelling
abdominal tenderness
abnormal growths
abnormal tissue formations
abscess
acid reflux
agitation
allergies
anemia
anxiety
bacterial infection
bactcrial overgrowths
bad breath (chronic)
bald spots
belching (chronic)
bloating
blood in stools
blood in urine
blood-shot eyes
body aches
body temperature fluctuations
bowel problems
breath issues
brittle bones
brittle hair
brittle nails
bruising
bulging eyes
bulging veins
burning pain
burping (chronic)
cataracts
chills
chronic anxiety
chronic bloating

chronic constipation
chronic depression
chronic diarrhea
chronic headache
chronic insomnia
chronic migraine
chronic nausea chronic
pain circulation issues
cloudy urine
cold feet
cold hands
cold sores
confusion
constipation
curved spine
decreased appetite
depression
diarrhea
difficulty concentrating
difficulty swallowing
digestive problems
disk degeneration
dizziness
drooping eyelids
drowsiness
dry eyes
dry mouth
ear issues
ear pain
enlarged glandes
enlarged veins
erectile dysfunction
excess gas
exhaustion
eye issues

Common Autoimmune Symptoms List (continued)

fainting
fatigue
fevers (reoccurring)
fistula
flatulence (excess)
food allergies
fullness in throat
fungal infections
fungus issues
gland or lymph problems
growths
gum issues
hair loss
hard spots
headache
hearing loss
heart burn
heart palpitations
heart problems
heartburn (chronic)
hemorrhoids
high blood pressure
high blood sugar levels
high cholesterol
hip issues
hives
hormonal imbalances
immune problems
indigestion
infections
inflammation (general)
insomnia
intestinal bleeding
intestinal obstruction
irregular heartbeat
irritability

itching (chronic)
jaw issues
jaw stiffness
joint inflammation
joint pain
light headedness
loss of muscle tone
low blood sugar levels
lumps
macular degeneration
memory issues
memory loss
menstrual problems
migraines
missed periods
mold issues
mood swings
muscle cramps
muscle hardness
muscle loss
muscle tightness
nail bed issues
nasal inflammation
nasal issues
nausea
nerve pain
nervousness
night sweats
numbness
organ failure
organ issues
ovarian cysts
overactive bladder
painful urination
parasite infections
polyps

Common Autoimmune Symptoms List (continued)

rapid heart beat
rashes
rectal bleeding
ringing in the ears
sensitivities
shaking
shortness of breath
skin discoloration
skin disorders
skin issues
skin rashes
skin spots
sleep issues
sore throat (chronic)
sorcs
stiffness
stomach problems
sweating (excessive)
swelling
swelling tissues
taste issues
tenderness
testicular pain
tingling

tissue degeneration
tongue issues
tooth issues (chronic)
twitching
ulcers
vaginal issues
viral infections
vision loss
vomiting (chronic)
weakness
weight gain
weight loss
white tongue
wrist pain
yeast infections
yellow eyes

The COVID-19 Charade

The worldwide pandemic, known as Corona Virus or COVID-19 has effectively shut down the world in terms of health/wellness, but also economy, lifestyle, transportation and the basic necessities such as being able to have a job or business, and the essentials of life.

Although there is much unknown about this invisible killer, common sense tells us that bolstering our immune function against viruses would be a prudent first step.

The response from our governmental "doctors in charge" has been questionable at best. No solid mention of immune support. Not unlike the traditional medical system's perspective and approach to autoimmunity, they seem to purposely avoid the published science, and common sense, when it comes to the COVID-19 virus as well. Could this be an effort to keep the public locked down and waiting for the trillion-dollar vaccine as their only hope to avoid succumbing to the virus?

For decades we have been in possession of solid anti-viral research in regard to natural immune modulators and other phytonutrients. Studies have demonstrated the modulators to inhibit the replication of viruses of many types including Newcastle disease virus (NDV), human immunodeficiency virus type 1 (HIV-1), infectious bursal disease virus (IBDV), infectious bronchitis virus, feline leukemia virus, H1N1 subtype influenza virus, and herpes simplex virus to name a few. Unless you are in the habit of studying scientific literature, it is highly unlikely that you have heard this before. The news reports nothing of interest if it is anti-pharmaceutical.

Given the science and information available, an answer to avoiding a viral take-over of the body could not be more clear; Restore strong and accurate immune function to the body.

The CDC tells us that *"older adults"* and people with *"Certain Medical Conditions"* are "the People at Increased Risk for Severe Illness" from COVID-19.

On their website under Certain Medical Conditions they list a slew of immune-suppression and autoimmune diseases, **without ever mentioning the words immune-suppression or autoimmunity.**

Short of dancing and singing, they seem to be doing everything in their power to avoid simply stating that **people with weak immune systems have difficulty fighting off COVID-19 (and viruses in general), therefore it would be wise to restore strong and accurate immune response.**

Notice, there is no mention of a correlation to declining immune response in their statement to follow:

The CDC (Centers for Disease Control): *"As you get older, your risk for severe illness from COVID-19 increases. For example, people in their 50s are at higher risk for severe illness than people in their 40s. Similarly, people in their 60s or 70s are, in general, at higher risk for severe illness than people in their 50s. The greatest risk for severe illness from COVID-19 is among those aged 85 or older."*

The NIAID (National Institutes of Allergy and Infectious Diseases) and the JCI (The Journal of Clinical Investigation) state the known consensus; *"The Immune System Declines with Age. The effects of aging on the immune system are manifest at multiple levels that include reduced production of B and T cells in bone marrow and thymus and diminished function of mature lymphocytes in secondary lymphoid tissues. As a result, elderly individuals do not respond to immune challenge as robustly as the young."*

Obviously, this is why the very young rarely die from the viral infection while a large percentage of the elderly succumb to the virus.

Investigating the obvious, researchers at the Barnes-Jewish Hospital and Missouri Baptist Medical Center in St. Louis, found that COVID-19 patients often had far fewer circulating immune cells than is typical. Further, the immune cells that were present did not secrete normal levels of cytokines (No surprise here). Cytokines are critical cell-signaling molecules that aid cell to cell communication in immune responses and stimulate the movement of cells towards sites of inflammation, infection and trauma.

We have witnessed Dr. Anthony Fauci, director of the National Institute of Allergy and Infectious Diseases (NIAID) step to the podium on numerous occasions during this COVID-19 pandemic. He has repeatedly instructed the public to wash their hands, ware masks (even googles), social distance, isolate, and in a multitude of different ways wait for the miracle vaccine.

Yet never once have we heard Dr. Fauci advise the public of the science published within his own Institute (the NIAID) concerning declining and weakened immunity as it relates to COVID deaths, the science, and common sense behind supporting the immune system in these challenging times, or any time for that matter. It is almost as if he views strong immune response as a *competitor* to the coming vaccine.

It is more than Wise to Armor Oneself

Why do people die from COVID-19? In short, because their immune systems can not overcome the virus, and subsequently, the virus overcomes the body. As stated above, their immune systems are producing reduced levels of B and T cells in bone marrow and thymus and diminished function of mature lymphocytes in secondary lymphoid tissues.

The immune modulating components, and in particular, Acemannan holds a major key to improved immune function. Acemannan is a polydispersed ßeta-(1, 4)-linked acetylated mannan with antiviral, antibacterial, and antifungal properties. It is an immunomodulator shown to cause the activation of immune macrophages and antibodies. It acts to stimulate the cytotoxic activity of natural killer T-cells and the generation of cytotoxic T-lymphocytes-mediated responses (CTLs). They significantly increase levels of B and T cells.

Simultaneously, stabilized immune modulators do not promote a cytokine storm. Science demonstrates that immune modulating cytokines, IL-10 for example, are produced by taking them. IL-10 is an example of an immune modulating Cytokine. It down regulates IL-1, IL-2 and IL-6 which are all pro inflammatory cytokines.

.Now we can not claim that the immune modulating components are a cure for COVID-19. But at this juncture, who in their right mind would argue that improved immune function, at all stages, would not be an ace in one's hand for winning the battle against the virus?

Additionally, physicians using the immune modulating components are reporting that patients who test positive for COVID, very rarely if ever need to go to the hospital if they have been on the immune modulators for varying periods of months. This has been our experience as well.

Where do these Immune Modulating Components come from?

It is the inner gel from a cultured Aloe vera Barbadensis leaf which contains the extraordinary healing components which are discussed in this book. Comparatively in regard to weight, these miraculous components exist in a very small proportion compared to the total weight of the plant.

Aloe vera gel from the leaf is 99.5% water by weight. The desirable healing components are found within the remaining 0.5.% (one-half of one percent) of the gel. Aloe vera juice is significantly more diluted and subsequently less potent. Both are unstabilized liquids, and over time will further lose what little proportional potency they possessed from the day of harvest.

A human being cannot physically ingest large quantities of Aloe gel or juice daily, in an attempt to ingest potency. Attempting to ingest enough Aloe gel or juice to render a significant healing effect will result in diarrhea from the aloin content, and a fullness in the intestinal tract which reduces appetite for solid food and additional nutrients.

The 0.5.% (one-half of one percent) healing component content must be extracted from the gel, stabilized and concentrated in order to produce a substance suitable for ingestion, and potent enough to exhibit significant healing benefit in a reasonable amount of time. The solution is the stabilized, concentrated extract from a cultured Aloe botanical which has produced the healing time frames against chronic diseases outlined above (AUTOIMMUNE-X). It contains stabilized concentrated immune modulating components primarily consisting of mannans, polymannans, polysaccharides, Acemannan, and multiple added healing co-factors form the plant, minus the plant irritants such as aloin.

Chapter 2

Anti-Aging
and
Cell Regeneration

Most people would prefer to live a youthful, productive, long and healthy life. The good news is that we can extend life and most importantly, improve the quality of life.

First and foremost, we must avoid cellular disease. We cannot feel and look young, strong and beautiful while struggling with disease. Avoidance of severe acute bacterial and viral diseases such as methacillin resistant staphylococcus aureus, E. coli, influenza, and the latest COVID-19 virus would save thousands of lives each year.

Lowering the risk of chronic degenerative diseases can increase the likelihood of a longer life. So the first way we can extend life expectancy and the quality of life is through *prevention,* and thus the avoidance of chronic diseases. Research on, and use of phytonutrients, and in particular immune modulating components, has demonstrated beneficial effects against a multitude of chronic and degenerative diseases.

Secondly, we must create a climate conducive to extending cell-life between divisions, and the number of times a cell may replicate. Both these feats of health and youth preservation can be accomplished through avoidance of disease and comprehensive cellular support through the ingestion of these specific phytonutrients.

Science has discovered that vital nutrients regulate RNA/DNA gene expression and cell life span!

Within the nucleus of the cell exists our genetic material, DNA *(Deoxyribonucleic acid)* which is the chemical "blueprint or master plan" for the cell. This genetic blueprint encodes information required for all life processes including growth, development and reproduction.

DNA is organized on string-like structures called chromosomes which contain our genes. Each gene contains the instructions to make a certain protein. The DNA directs the formation of RNA *(ribonucleic acid)*. All within the cell, the RNA moves out of the nucleus into the cytoplasm and enters the ribosome where the specific protein called for by the RNA is assembled according to the amino acid code.

DNA is made up of four specific amino acids called adenine, cytosine, guanine, and thiamine. These are generally referred to by their initials A, C, G, and T. They are strung together in various combinations to form individual genes which have specific functions.

The function of a gene is to produce strands of messenger ribonucleic acid called mRNA. This process is known as *"gene expression."* mRNA is made of the chemical bases A, C, G, and uracil (U) instead of thiamine (T).

Individual mRNAs then are used to string various amino acids together to make specific proteins, (RNAs) which run the different body functions. In other words, *gene expression* is the process in which the genetic code within the DNA is deciphered to produce a functional protein or RNA. A functional protein, for example, could be a structural protein such as collagen, or an important functional hormone such as insulin, testosterone, estrogen, or progesterone.

When toxins are present or required nutrients are missing, mistakes are made in gene expression, and thus the accurate replication of

DNA. These mistakes can result in whole sections of the DNA being left out or just a single letter at a specific place being changed from one to another. This then leads to mistakes in how the amino acids are aligned in a protein. This can then affect the function of the protein leading to a particular disease, usually and often times inappropriately referred to as a *"genetic"* disease. These mistakes can be passed on to future generations of cells as well as future generations of offspring.

Without proper DNA replication through gene expression, cellular growth, tissue repair, reproduction and hormone production, to name a few of the vital physiological processes, are inhibited or cannot occur. The cellular demand for nutrients is critical and can vary as a function of growth, development, age, reproductive status, and immunity. Certain nutrients also play critical informational or signaling roles in cellular communication.

The expression of genes involved in nutrient storage, processing, and metabolism can be influenced by the cell's nutrient environment. Gene expression is promoted or constrained by the quality of the nutrient environment. Therefore, deficiencies in any necessary nutrient have direct negative impacts on cellular health.

Of all the critical functions that could be discussed in relation to nutrient support of the cells and the body, no area of nutritional need could be more critical than the support of RNA/DNA gene expression in combating premature aging and disease. If there is a fountain of youth and health within the body, it is the accurate and continuous reproduction of this gene expression in which vital nutrients play the pivotal role.

Each cell can replicate itself by its ability to divide and multiply. In cellular reproduction, a gene carries biological information in a form which must be accurately copied and then transmitted from each cell to all its genetic cellular descendants.

Situated at the ends of DNA strands are *telomeres*. These molecules program the replication of new cells. Telomeres are responsible for cellular reproduction. Telomeres perform a function in aligning the DNA molecule during replication, keeping it from being copied out of synch. The molecular length of these telomeres determines how many cell divisions remain before the cell will die. Each time the cell replicates, a little bit of the telomere is lost, so that eventually when the telomere length is exhausted, the cell can no longer replicate itself and will subsequently die. The number of potential replications has been discovered to vary between 40 and 90, depending on cell type, and is known as the *"Hayflick number,"* after Leonard Hayflick who discovered this phenomenon in 1965.

The miracle of *cell division* (replication) is the process in which a cell divides (splits or duplicates) into two new cells. Cell division is the basis of all perpetuating life forms. Each time our cells duplicate themselves, the DNA molecule, which resembles a spiral ladder or *"helix,"* splits along the "rungs" of the ladder. Each half then rebuilds the missing half making two new DNA molecules. The two new cells thus created are nearly identical to the parent cell (which no longer *exists*), except the two new cell's DNA possess slightly shorter telomeres. The quality of the new cells formed is dependent upon the availability of the vital nutrients present. Poor quality or lack of vital nutrient components adversely affect the new cells just created.

Optimally, the anti-aging goal is to support the health of the cell, extend cell-life between replications, while avoiding disease in order to experience the full potential of the telomeres ability to replicate. Lowering the risk of chronic degenerative diseases enables the cell to live out its full telomere potential. Cells which are not receiving adequate nutritional support may become diseased or die long before their telomere potential has been exhausted.

The human body was designed to continually regenerate itself and to replicate new cells that must replace the old, making as exact a copy as possible. For the new cells thus created to be healthy and to replicate as accurately as possible, thus slowing the aging process, all healing components and essential nutrients must be present. Imperfect cell reproduction leads to premature aging and chronic degenerative disease.

The efficiency of DNA repair depends to a great extent on numerous healing components and essential nutrients being available on a continuous basis. When a new liver, heart, stomach, or immune system cell needs to be replicated, there is no time to waste. These essential components must be present at all times. Without them we suffer cellular damage, age prematurely, and are susceptible to widespread diseases.

Why has this information been kept on the sidelines while we play SRR (Symptom Relief Roulette)?

"The Cell is Immortal"

Many scientists studying mortality now believe that *aging itself is really **a dis-ease,*** and not the inevitable experience of the biological organism. In other words, the rate of aging is not our predetermined fate!

French scientist, Dr. Alexis Carrel, received the Nobel Prize for keeping the cells of a chicken heart alive for 34 years. Dr. Carrel concluded: ***"The cell is immortal. It is merely the fluid in which it floats that degenerates. Renew this fluid at intervals, give the cells what they require for nutrition, and as far as we know, the pulsation of life may go on forever."***

After studying his research, we believe what Dr. Alexis Carrel was stating, and we certainly concur: ***"If the cell can be maintained in an optimum state of support, lacking nothing within its nutrient-rich, contaminate-free intracellular and extracellular fluids, then theoretically, it could continue to replicate and live forever. Moreover, and notwithstanding the immortal concept, but most certainly, if one's cells are maintained in an optimum state of support, lacking nothing within their nutrient-rich, contaminate- free intracellular and extracellular fluids, then they will indeed resist disease, live significantly longer, and without any doubt, provide a higher quality of life along the way."***

Currently, a large body of scientific research documented on four continents including two studies from Harvard University researchers, has been successful in demonstrating significantly extended healthy cell-life with the use of natural phytonutrients such as polyphenols and flavones. In one study, polyphenols were shown to initiate a genetic mechanism known to protect mice against the degenerative diseases of aging and prolonged their life spans by thirty percent. In another study the life span of yeast cells was increased by sixty to eighty percent. Meanwhile, the information is being sidelined while drug patents have been apparently filed under the guise of *"revisions of the natural molecules."* Fortunately we can ingest these wonderful phytonutrients now, in their natural form and design as intended, rather than wait for a pharmaceutical firm to alter the natural molecules and create something *"revised,"* which may injure or potentially kill us.

Three major physiologic factors in the aging process are:

1. Cellular starvation due to the lack of specific vital nutrients and/or sub-optimal digestive function.
2. Cellular dehydration (lack of sufficient extracellular and intracellular fluids)
3. Toxin-related cellular damage (including RNA/DNA damage)

How to effectively combat aging (and disease), *simplified*

(1). Insure the daily maintenance of the digestive tract, the doorway to health, disease prevention, and recovery. **(immune modulating components)**

(2). Consuming Quality not Quantity: Consume a nutrient-dense diet, including phytonutrient, vitamin and mineral supplements, while minimizing your total caloric intake to maintain your optimum body weight. (See "Food Recommendations for Optimum Health, page 109).

(3). Insure Adequate Hydration: Drink 6, 8-ounce. glasses of water for a sedentary person, and 8 to 10 ounce glasses of water (or more) for the more active. (See "Food Recommendations for Optimum Health, page 109).

(4). Avoid toxins and synthetics (See "Slow Death List," page 107).

(5). Avoid stress whenever possible (See page 83).

(6). Exercise daily (See you doctor for potential restrictions).

(7). Receive fresh air and moderate sunshine daily when possible. (See, "Here Comes the Sun," page 119).

So as we can see, combating aging is not so complex. It involves ingesting what we are designed for, avoiding what we are not designed for and what hurts us, and doing what helps us.

The Alkaline Environment
Critical points that must be understood

The health of a cell, its ability to replicate, communicate, and subsequently our overall health in general depend on the delivery of adequate amounts of vital nutrients to the cell. Equally as important, the environment (extracellular fluid) in which the cell is operating must be conducive or friendly to the promotion of health, and unfriendly to the development and proliferation of disease. Diseases thrive in an acidic, low oxygen environment. A mild alkaline pH solution has available over 100 times as much oxygen as a mild acidic solution. Diseases do not thrive in such an environment.

Why has this information been kept on the sidelines?

The normal pH range of the blood is between 7.35 and 7.45 with the optimum pH level being approximately 7.4. This blood pH level of 7.4 is so important for the optimum health of the cells and subsequently the entire body. The body possesses buffering systems that strive to ensure the maintenance of this pH level. When nutrient deficiencies occur, causing the blood pH to fall below the optimum level, the body will begin to pull calcium and other pH buffering agents from the tissues and other areas of the body such as the bones, leading to osteoporosis. The body will take these desperate measures depleting other areas of calcium and essential nutrients in order to maintain the optimum blood pH.

If your body is forced to pull calcium and other essential nutrients from any other part of the body to supply the blood, this causes depletion of those essential nutrients from those areas, potentially leading to degenerative disease.

Unless you are ingesting sufficient amounts of minerals including calcium, it is impossible for your body to maintain optimum pH levels. If these deficiencies of minerals and calcium persist over an extended period of time, you have the biochemical basis or biological environment for premature aging and chronic degenerative disease.

In line with the concept of "the biological terrain," (discussed on page 129), diseases do not thrive or spread in an oxygen-rich, alkaline extracellular environment. Some of the most powerful disease-causing bacteria are anaerobic organisms which thrive in an oxygen poor environment. Adequate oxygen levels present in the blood and cellular fluids prohibit these harmful bacteria from surviving.

Cancer cell metabolism is a fermentation process that does not require free oxygen. Fermentation is a process of cellular energy production in an anaerobic environment (with reduced oxygen present). In an alkaline environment with the presence of adequate oxygen levels fermentation does not occur. Anaerobic metabolism's by-product is acid.

All cells and tissues depend on an alkaline environment containing an adequate supply of oxygen. The main reason poor circulation is such a problem, is because of the cellular damage it causes due to the lack of oxygen delivered to the tissues. In a heart attack or stroke for instance, the cells of the heart or brain die due to a lack of oxygen.

An alkaline environment of 7.4 is ideal for optimum health. Based on numerous studies, Immune modulating components, numerous phytonutrients, most minerals, and particularly calcium have a buffering or alkalizing effect on the body. In other words, they reduce the excess acidity of the body.

Aside from The Establishment's misinformation campaign, how did we slip into this age of disease? In short, mineral and nutrient deficiencies promote lower pH average values, higher acidity, lower levels of cellular function and communication, and higher levels of disease and deterioration. The aging process is accelerated and the life-span shortened.

"Every degenerative disease can be traced back to an organic mineral deficiency." Two time Nobel Prize winner, Linus Pauling.

In summary, by receiving sufficient mineral and specific nutrient intake, thus improving cellular function, communication, and raising pH values of the cell environment to an alkaline 7.4, the risk of disease can be dramatically reduced or altogether eliminated. Aging is generally characterized by the declining ability to respond to stress, increasing homeostatic imbalance, and increased risk of disease. Because of this, death is the ultimate consequence of aging. The efficiency of DNA repair, antioxidant enzymes, and rates of free radical production, all relate to aging and life expectancy. It has been determined that DNA damage can occur due to toxins and damage due to free radicals. Many phytonutrients, and in particular calcium and immune modulating components have been shown to support the extracellular alkaline environment, reduce the levels of toxins from disease causing organisms, have antioxidant (free radical protective) functions, and possess anti-inflammatory properties (inflammation is a major factor in all degenerative disease). These natural components have normalizing, homeostatic, and balancing effects on the gastrointestinal, sugar regulatory, and immune systems, supporting health, anti-aging, and longevity.

Addressing Stress

Stress cannot be overlooked when discussing anti-aging and overall health. Stress continues to be one of the leading players in the propagation and proliferation of physical and psychological illness.

Research has revealed that 65 to 90% of illness is stress-*related*. The very subject would prove to be tedious and time-consuming to break down in terms of types of stress and how they are manifested, so the most prudent approach would be to target the ailments that have been aforementioned in this book.

An important intracellular connection to alleviating and quite possibly preventing some of the most disastrous conditions may lie, to a good degree, in what we understand about our physical, social and environmental triggers that surround us every second of every day. Whether the stress arises from daily pressures to any variety of frustrations, jeopardy to our overall wellness may lie in the balance.

Let it never be said that we are not the "drivers of the bus." In many ways, the control of our own wellbeing is a function of how we manage our lives, loves, and passions. These can be positive or negative. It is all in the perception. One way or another, if left unbridled, stress can acutely or chronically devastate our state of overall wellness. Mental stress is known to be responsible for aggravating and contributing to the cause of many diseases. Heart disease, digestive disorders, arthritis, and diabetes encompass just a few. Although it is clear that stress alone does not cause these conditions, it is also clear that these and many other illnesses are influenced negatively by stress.

According to the National Institute of Mental Health (NIMH), an estimated 26.2% of Americans 18 and older suffer from a diagnosable mental disorder in a given year. Apply to this the 2004 census, and the translation is a staggering 57.7 million people. Mental disorders are the leading cause of disability in the U.S. and Canada for ages 15-44. It stands to reason and is backed by sound statistics that many suffer from more than one condition at a time. Approximately half of those with any mental disorder meet the criteria for 2 or more disorders, with severity strongly related to this fact. The remainder of mood and anxiety disorders alone approaches 150 million adults.

Stress is increased under such circumstances as injury, infection, surgery, chronic or acute illness, or with psychological stress. Psychological stress can presumably interfere with every physiologic function including digestion, and cause lack of sleep, fatigue, weight loss or gain. Stress increases the need for essential nutrients of all types such as protein, complex carbohydrates, essential fatty acids, vitamins and minerals. Conversely, the *lack* of sufficient nutrition in general, is known to elevate both physical and psychological stress.

Enough with the stress . . . now let us talk about *The Code!*

Note: *Some within the scientific community have utilized the term "The Code of Life" to metaphorically describe the predetermined genetic codes within the DNA strands.*

This book; "The Code of Life..." focuses on the hidden symbolized language which cells utilize to communicate with each other and the immune system, which ultimately supports every physiological function within the body including proper DNA replication. The human body, composed of matter and interacting energy, operates via these coded systems. Both metaphoric uses of the term are correct and only differ regarding the areas of coding being studied."

Chapter 3

The Code of Life

We now begin our journey into the most amazing health revelation ever discovered. *"The Code of Life"* operating within us should be understood by all. The wonderful news is that we can all benefit from this astounding discovery.

Although the science can be complex at times, we will speak in simplified terms initially, until the basic concept can be grasped. Further scientific exploration will follow as the chapters progress.

Cellular Communication

For decades, scientists in the field of biochemistry and cellular communication have attempted to break the biological code which enables the trillions of cells that make up our bodies to communicate with each other. This communication between cells is vital for virtually every system, structure, and function within the body. This is *"The Code of Life."*

Briefly, these physiological functions include the formation of collagen for bone, muscle and skin, the support and self-regulation of blood sugar levels, the maintenance of proper digestive function, the regulation and control of inflammatory processes, and proper immune system modulation.

Collagen is essential for proper wound healing and tissue formation. In fact, collagen makes up more than 25% of the total protein content of our body. Blood sugar levels are critical for cardiovascular health, brain function, and metabolism. Optimum digestive function is of dire necessity to ensure the delivery of an adequate supply of vital nutrients to every single cell in our bodies. The regulation of inflammation is essential for wound healing and tissue formation, and left unchecked is a major risk factor for a multitude of chronic diseases including arthritis, heart disease, and cancer.

As stated, this cellular communication is also vital for proper immune system modulation. It involves the identification of foreign invaders and the exchange of information necessary to maintain the health of each individual cell making up every tissue and organ of our bodies. Cellular communication is the very foundation of health. When this communication breaks down or becomes hindered, auto-immune disease (self-attacking-self), premature aging, and a multitude of system malfunctions are likely to arise throughout the body.

A Perspective on "Disease"

For the last century and a half, the *traditional medical community's* approach to disease has been based upon the *"germ theory."* This theory states that disease is caused by exposure to pathogenic organisms from the environment, without emphasis to the body's environmental state of health. The traditional medical community also insists that many diseases are *"incurable."* In other words, they are stating that the altered function and *"lack of ease"* (dis-ease) associated with the particular labeled condition is non-reversible, or that at least they do not understand how to restore the *"ease"* to the bodily functions which would eradicate the *cause* of the condition. This mentality is expressed in the drug-based approach of treating symptoms rather than addressing and correcting the root cause or causes. *Symptoms* are the body's warning signals of trouble from within. Taking a medication designed to simply suppress the symptoms of a disease without addressing the root cause, could be likened to turning off the fire alarm while your house burns. Adding fuel to the flames are the unavoidable side effects and toxicity of most pharmaceutical medications.

In contrast to the *germ theory* is the understanding of "The Biological Terrain" (page 129). This understanding is based upon the fact that if the body is maintained in a healthy state, it remains more resistant to disease regardless of exposure to potential disease-causing organisms. (More on The Biological Terrain in Chapter 5).

Look at the word "disease" from a different perspective: Webster's definition of disease: *Lack of ease; uneasiness; trouble; an alteration in the state of the body or of some of its organs interrupting or disturbing the performance of the vital functions and causing or threatening pain and weakness; malady; affliction; illness; sickness; and disorder. ...etc.*

What did we just read? Condensed;

"Dis-ease" is "trouble" - an alteration in the state of the body. . . *interrupting or disturbing* the performance...etc.

A body existing in a state of *"ease,"* is one receiving all vital nutritional components, whose cells are communicating (sharing vital information), and whose organs are performing all vital functions unencumbered. Conversely, *"dis-ease"* is a lack of *"ease."* It occurs within the body when there is confusion or disruption due to miscommunication or a lack of needed components.

Science has revealed that when vital nutrients are not available, cells miscommunicate. When cells miscommunicate, breakdowns occur in the structure and functions of the defense and healing processes. Nutrients are not delivered to cells requiring them. Harmful invaders entering the body are not efficiently eliminated and are left unchecked to wreak havoc. Generally speaking, when the body is supplied with all vital nutritional components, and when cells are communicating efficiently, there exists an *"ease"* or an *optimum state of health.* When cells lack vital nutrients or components, causing miscommunication, we have the potential for a state of acute or chronic dis-ease.

This being fact, if you presently have some sort of disorder or disease, your focus should be to return your body to a state of *ease* in order to reduce the disorder or confusion within. The reader presently following this line of logic may be getting somewhat excited and asking the following question:

"Well, does this mean that if I return my body to a state of "ease" that I can cure myself of any disease that I am presently afflicted with?"

As stated previously, with this healing process being described, we and scores of our colleagues have witnessed patients dramatically improve, and in most cases, literally walk away from diseases altogether, most of which the traditional medical community labels as "incurable" (they label all autoimmune diseases as incurable). For our purposes now, we will state that we firmly believe from our shared experiences and from the analysis of hundreds of research studies from around the world, that the very first step to prevention and recovery from existing disease is to bring the body into a state of overall ease, enabling the body's innate and complex healing mechanisms to function effectively and as designed. Briefly for now, this is accomplished by supplying the body with the key vital nutrients and healing components it requires, while avoiding harmful substances and making a firm effort to reduce psychological stress.

Interestingly, it has been documented that malignant (cancer) cells often display incomplete or abnormal sugars (communicators) on their surfaces. In other words, cellular recognition and communication has been disrupted in these cells.

Efficient cellular communication throughout the body will promote an ideal state of ease throughout the body. The more efficiently the process of cellular communication is allowed to function, the greater the effect of preventing and overcoming existing disease. This explains why so many researchers worldwide, addressing such a wide variety of biological processes as well as diseases, have demonstrated highly favorable results when the basic components of what we refer to as the "symbols" (specific vital nutrients) of *The Code of Life* are provided. These specific vital nutrients are abundant in high concentration within the immune modulating components.

Second Note to the Reader

A brief discussion of terms follows. We would like to emphasize that the reader need not be intimidated by the terms used periodically throughout this book. It is not necessary to memorize them. Many of these terms are used interchangeably by scientists, such as; Complex carbohydrates, polysaccharides, polymannans, Acemannan, Healing Orchestrators, and Conductor Molecules. <u>All of these are Immune Modulating Components.</u> All of these are complex carbohydrates and depending on the molecular weight (Dalton) of each, they can be interchangeable terms, one the same as the other.

The inner gel of the Aloe vera Barbadensis Miller plant consists of a wide variety of phytonutrients and healing components (200 plus determined to date). These include but are not limited to; vitamins, minerals, enzymes, lignins, plant sterols, fatty acids, salicylic acid, amino acids, and most importantly the complex carbohydrate molecules known as polymannans and polysaccharides, which are also known as "The Healing Orchestrators," and "Conductor Molecules." These complex carbohydrates are the immune modulating components.

Polymannans are complex carbohydrates which are made up of individual *"sugar"* molecules linked together to form molecular chains of various lengths. **These complex *"sugars"* are not sugar as we think of table sugar. They do not increase blood sugar levels, but in fact help to normalize blood sugar levels.** They are not used by the body for their caloric content; rather, they are incorporated into cells, cell membranes, antibodies, hormones, connective tissues, and many other vital functional areas of the body. (For further explanation see *The Difference Between Simple and Complex Sugars* Page 162)

Researchers have concluded that the very long-chain polymannans of one million Dalton and greater (Acemannan), help orchestrate the other healing components of the Aloe Healing Orchestra and they have thus been named "The Healing Orchestrators," or "Conductor Molecules." They are one in the same. (Dalton is a unit of mass used in physics and chemistry).

Curiously, the root of "mannose" is manna, which the Bible records as the food God supplied to the Israelites for their survival during their journey through the Sinai Peninsula. "The people ground it, or pounded it, and then baked it (Num. 11:8). A double portion was to be found on the day before the Sabbath, when none was to be found."

In our practices and subsequently our research, we have found mannose containing stabilized polymannans to contain The Code of Life. We find it intriguing that according to the bible, mannose was the food of choice sent by God for the survival of the people.

Tracking down the Code

Biochemistry is the chemistry of life. It is the scientific study of the chemistry of living cells, tissues, organs, and organisms. It is the study of the processes occurring within the living cell. Humans are composed of trillions of cells, most cannot be seen by the naked eye. For decades, biochemists have attempted to break the biological code by which the cells of the body communicate with one another. This communication between cells allows the multitude of vital processes of the body to occur. This is the complex physiological method of communication referred to here as The Code   of   Life.

The major classes of biomolecules are proteins, including nucleic acids, lipids (fats), and carbohydrates. Until recently, scientists focused on proteins as the primary molecules of communication between cells. Protein molecules were believed to perform most if not all of the basic biological processes necessary for cells to communicate. The importance of carbohydrates had been mainly ignored due to the fact that carbohydrates were considered to be only a source of calories. Considering the fact that there are many more molecular configurations possible with carbohydrate molecules as compared to proteins, researchers began to suspect that carbohydrates were actually the primary molecules of cellular communication.

The July 2002 issue of Scientific American stated: *"In contrast, the roughly 10 simple sugars common in mammalian carbohydrates can join with one another at many different points and can form intricate branching structures. Moreover, two linked units do not always orient the same way: sometimes a building block will point up relative to another unit, and sometimes it will point down.*

In contrast, the four nucleotides in the DNA "alphabet" can combine to produce 256 different four-unit structures, and the 20 amino acids in proteins can yield about 16,000 four-unit configurations. But the simplest sugars (the carbohydrates, ED.) in the body can theoretically assemble into more than 15 million four component arrangements. Although not all these combinations occur in nature, the possibilities remain overwhelming. "

These are the bulk of the "symbols" making up The Code.

We can clearly see from these comparisons the importance of these complex carbohydrate and subsequently these simple sugar molecules in regard to cellular communication. In addition, to work effectively, certain therapeutic proteins must have particular sugars attached to them at precise sites.

Despite the fact that the human body can breakdown complex carbohydrates (polymannans) into simple sugars and can then reassemble them into more complex structures, the body cannot produce the vital polymannans in their various forms. They are essential and the body must have them for the prevention of disease and optimum health.

Utilizing newly developed analytical techniques permitting the investigation of these biologically active phytonutrients, it has been recently determined that not only are there thousands of different carbohydrate molecules, but many of them can take multiple forms to accomplish different tasks.

These innumerable carbohydrate (polysaccharide) molecules possess virtually limitless flexibility to perform a multitude of different functions throughout the body. Fortunately, due to the fact that there are many more molecular configurations possible with polysaccharides as compared to proteins, it became logical to investigate these carbohydrates as possibly being the basis, in large, of the biological information (the symbols of the Code). In large, they actually make up the physiological Code which determines the endless functions that must be carried out on a moment to moment, minute by minute, and hour by hour basis, over our entire lifetime.

Many of these processes of communication, previously assumed to be performed by protein molecules, are actually performed by a wide variety of complex carbohydrate molecules including; polymannans, polysaccharides, glycoproteins, glycolipids, glucomannans, and others. These precisely shaped molecules attach to and protrude from cell surfaces and are recognized and understood by neighboring cells.

The polysaccharide molecules are involved vastly in cellular recognition, including immune functions. Without these complex carbohydrates that attach to cell surfaces, the body's operating systems can break down, resulting in an entire host of disorders, immune and autoimmune diseases which either weaken or inactivate their normal response, or cause immune cells to attack and destroy our healthy tissues. Without them, our disease-fighting cells may not recognize disease-causing invaders such as bacteria, viruses, fungi, parasites, toxins, or even cancer cells. Hormones may be misdirected, contributing to physical and emotional problems, and pre-mature aging. It is an undisputed fact that health begins at the cellular level. Interestingly, most if not all of the building blocks of these biologically active carbohydrates, as well as many unique healing carbohydrate compounds, are found in high concentrations within one plant.

The Miracle Plant

To fully appreciate the incredible healing properties and potentials of the Aloe-derived polymannans and other healing components, we must understand how they function. Fortunately, due to a great increase in interest in this field, recent research has shed much light.

How can it be that so many compounds contained within one plant can be so helpful for so many illnesses, including cancer, diabetes, arthritis, colitis, ulcerative colitis, irritable bowel syndrome, Crohn's disease, ulcers, GERD, psoriasis, wound healing, burns, infectious diseases, auto-immune diseases, etc.? The list is virtually endless.

Traditional biochemistry and nutrition has had a great interest in amino acids (building blocks of proteins), lipids and fats (building blocks of hormones), vitamins and minerals (essential catalysts which help produce energy), but again had little to say about polysaccharides except that they were burned for their caloric content. It was believed, even though no research ever proved it, that these complex carbohydrates were broken down to the simple sugar, glucose, and that if needed, all the other polysaccharides could be built up from glucose alone. Once again, these complex "sugars" are not sugar as we think of table sugar. They do not increase blood sugar levels, but in fact help to normalize blood sugar levels.

Until recently, analytical techniques which biochemists utilized were inadequate to study these long-chain and very complex polymannan molecules. Research has shown that mannose, the major component of the Aloe-derived polymannan is taken up by liver cells for glycoprotein synthesis (vital for cellular communication) directly from mannose, NOT FROM GLUCOSE. The significance of this is that glucose is readily available in the diet but *mannose* is not. Glucose is readily available in our food supply and need not be supplemented. However, mannose, essential for its immune and communication function, among others, is all but missing from the modern-day food supply.

As previously discussed, there are quite possibly other reasons as well why these healing polysaccharides have been ignored for so long by mainstream medicine. In my opinion, this information has not been shared with the public for obvious financial reasons, including the tremendous loss of income the pharma/medical establishment would suffer if this information were better understood by the public. The fact that these Aloe-derived substances cannot be patented is most likely the major reason why the pharmaceutical industry has not been interested in sharing the news. Profits are based on treating the symptoms of illnesses with drugs and procedures, not providing cures, and certainly not natural, unpatentable cures.

For a multitude of reasons relating to improved health, the ingestion of these Aloe-derived polysaccharides is vitally important. The human digestive tract has cells called *endocytes* that actually take up these Aloe-derived substances intact.

It has been determined that after they are transported into the bloodstream, they are utilized as is or broken down and reassembled to form other compounds or "symbols."

Cellular communication is essential for virtually every important function in the body. How does the stomach know when and how much acid and digestive enzymes to produce? How do the killer cells of the immune system recognize your own healthy tissues from foreign invaders such as bacteria, viruses, fungi, parasites, or other disease-causing pathogens? How do our killer immune cells recognize a healthy cell from a diseased one such as a cancer cell? The answer is astounding!

On the surface of each cell are protein and carbohydrate molecules that miraculously identify through the code, the state of intracellular activity (within the cell). Other cells that must interact are also covered with their own protein and carbohydrate identifiers that determine how they will specifically interact with the others, and so on down the physiological line until the desired substance is produced and the desired effect is obtained.

This production line, controlled in large by these polysaccharide encoders is responsible for the formation of enzymes, hormones, neurotransmitters, substrates, and the building blocks of life. New cells, glands, tissues, organs, and re-growth and repair are carried out in this fashion. The symbols in this coded language are the key to these processes of growth, reproduction, regeneration, healing, cell repair, and recovery from disease. Improved function results from the restoration and adequate maintenance of this process.

It has been shown that even the ends of dendrites (extensions of nerve cells) are surrounded by immune cells, indicating that there exists cellular communication between the nervous and immune systems. These communications or chemical messages are often controlled by these carbohydrate-containing molecules. The process known as chemotaxis (the movement of cells controlled by chemical messengers) is to a great extent, dependent upon the symbols in this code. It has been determined that energy is required to convert these molecules from one form to another. Also, the rate of these conversions is dependent on the quantities of these molecules present. The greater the presence, the faster the rate of production. It is scientifically apparent that sub-essential communication between cells, and between cells and the immune system causes us to age prematurely, inevitably contract disease, and if lacking severely, cease to exist.

There is much current research being directed to more fully decipher this coded language. In the meantime, we can benefit enormously by ensuring adequate consumption of the building blocks of this code – the full compliment of Aloe-derived healing components including the short, medium, long, and very long chain polymannans, which are the components and building blocks, in conjunction with adequate protein, phytonutrient, mineral and vitamin support of which more will be discussed.

The dietary lack of these complex carbohydrates and nutrients will become recognized as a major deficiency syndrome. I have named this condition Cellular and Immune Communication Deficiency Syndrome (C.I.C.D.S). Just as many of the deficiency syndromes currently recognized today were misunderstood as to their origins, C.I.C.D.S. has been largely unidentified and yet will prove to be the underlying cause of a vast number of immune, auto-immune, and chronic degenerative diseases as well as premature aging.

Due to the absence of these essential polysaccharide phytonutrients and support components, including vitamins and minerals in our modern food supply, we all may be currently suffering from C.I.C.D.S to a greater or lesser degree. Soil depletion, pesticides, gene manipulation, hormones, toxins, pollution, processed, preserved, adulterated, fast and overcooked foods are but a few reasons for the gradual destruction of these vital natural compounds. These biologically active components possess numerous healing properties in addition to their cellular communication functions. They are essential to our quality of life and survival! They are our food and medicine by design.

Chapter 4

What Has Happened To Our Food?

As discussed in the introduction, the food we eat today is far removed from what our grandparents or great-grandparents ate. In those days, all food was "organically grown." There were no artificial fertilizers, pesticides, herbicides, hormones, antibiotics, or "genetically modified" food crops. Most food was grown locally and was consumed within a few days of being picked or caught. It was not sprayed with preservatives, mold inhibitors, or waxes. The soil was rich with nutrients and essential minerals yielding crops which were high in the same.

Healthy soil is a living environment containing nitrogen-fixing bacteria, minerals, and is alive with rich organic matter. A process known as "rotational farming" or "crop rotation" maintained the nutritional quality of the soil. This was accomplished by a particular crop being planted in a field one year, being plowed back into the earth, and then another crop planted the following year. Alfalfa, for example, would be planted because its root systems would absorb minerals deep from within the soil. It would then be plowed back into the soil and a new crop such as corn would be planted to reap the benefits from the newly revitalized soil. Some years the land was not planted at all and any organic waste was returned to the soil to decompose and allow its nutrients to be returned to it. Organic fertilizers such as manure, compost, and lime (for essential magnesium and alkalinity) were used. Organic soil requires bacteria that actually "fix" nitrogen, increasing the protein content of the food, and when bound to minerals these proteins form "chelated" organically bound minerals which are more easily absorbed.

Presently cattle, foul, (chicken, turkey, duck, Cornish hen, etc.) and even fish are being fed an unnatural diet of corn, antibiotics, growth hormones, pesticides, preservatives and artificial coloring agents. "Farm-raised" salmon are being fed a mix of corn, antibiotics, and other synthetic chemicals and coloring agents. These salmon do not possess nearly as much of the essential omega III fatty acids as wild caught salmon. A coloring agent is also added, which turns the grey colored salmon to a *"healthy looking"* orange color. Nevertheless, these salmon do not contain the naturally-occurring bright orange antioxidant plant pigments which provide many of the "wild caught" salmons' health benefits.

A steer has a normal diet of grass containing a healthy mix of essential fatty acids, amino acids, minerals, cellulose, fiber, chlorophyll, enzymes and other plant nutrients necessary for their proper health and development. They incorporate these essential nutrients and when we consume them we gain the benefits as well. When we consume artificially fed animals that have been raised consuming a mineral, essential fatty acid, and phytonutrient deficient diet of commercially produced grains, we become deficient as well. A prime example is the omega III to omega VI essential fatty acid ratio. Many authors have stated that this ratio should be 1:1 (one part omega III to one part omega VI) and no more than 1:3 (one part of omega III to three parts omega VI). Our modern diet has been estimated to be 1:20! In other words, we are not receiving nearly enough omega III essential fatty acids and we are consuming far too much omega VI containing oils. This essential fatty acid imbalance contributes to systemic inflammation, which increases the likelihood of stroke, heart attacks, arthritis, other inflammatory diseases and many other diseases including cancer.

Currently, mass produced food is being grown by a number of giant food corporations who routinely use artificial fertilizers containing only three ingredients: potassium, phosphorus, and nitrogen. The problem with these artificial fertilizers is that they do not contain any of the other innumerable substances that are contained in natural fertilizers such as minerals, nitrogen-fixing bacteria (essential for protein production), and numerous other vital components.

Furthermore, their use further depletes the soil of whatever nutrients it may contain and destroys its ability to grow plants which yield produce containing significant amounts of phytonutrients.

Crops grown with artificial fertilizers on depleted soils are far more prone to disease, insects and other pests, so pesticides, herbicides, and other poisonous sprays are routinely applied. This practice introduces additional toxins to these nutrient deficient foods. So not only are we consuming foods containing numerous poisonous chemicals, and which are severely lacking in nutritional value, but in addition, the components which make up *The Code of Life,* and all supporting phytonutrients in *The Universal Spectrum of Life* are largely absent!

"Hybridized" is defined as the interbreeding between two animals or plants. Hybridization may produce a desired quality such as increased sugar content or *"shelf life"* but at the same time may also *remove* naturally occurring nutrients that are of great importance.

The rearranging of the genetic plant material between populations or species is often called hybridization. Many, present company included, consider most hybridization an outrage on nature producing an unnatural product. Genetically modified foods may look good, stay "fresh" longer, and be sweeter, but lack essential vitamins, minerals, and phytonutrients such as antioxidants including; selenium, vitamin E, carotenoids, proanthocyanidans, chlorophyll, etc., as compared to unmodified organically grown natural produce. Genetic modification is the process of manipulating genes outside the organism's natural reproductive process. Hybridization matches two strands of DNA that were not originally paired. There exists a growing consensus that this process, which rarely and in some cases would never occur in nature, may have totally unpredictable consequences which we as a species may come to regret.

As reported recently, honeybee populations have been mysteriously disappearing. Bees are dying in such dramatic numbers that the economic consequences could soon be dire. Some experts believe that the large scale use of genetically modified plants, and in particular, pollen from genetically modified corn is the culprit. Albert Einstein, recognizing the vital link in nature and survival of all species which the bees support stated: *"If the bee disappears from the surface of the earth, man would have no more than four years to live. No more bees - no more pollination - no more men!"* We choose this example to make the illustration that there is no sacred ground that is immune from interference. Even areas of nature that are critical to our very survival are at risk by the hands of those who would experiment with our futures in the name of higher corporate profits.

Due to these unnatural procedures employed with the focus on mass production and cost reduction, in conjunction with the elimination of varieties of foods, our modern diet is lacking in the essential healing carbohydrates and other plant nutrients. Missing in particular are the long and very long chain polymannans, so important for the prevention and elimination of most of the chronic degenerative diseases that prevail and are continuing to increase.

Traditionally, herbalists and naturalists speak of the "bitter elements" that give organically and "wild harvested" herbs, fruits and vegetables their distinctive taste, smell and healing properties. I recall visiting a friend who had just returned from visiting relatives in Italy. Upon arrival to his home, I commented that his kitchen smelled of garlic. He showed me a garlic clove that he had brought back from Italy. I could actually smell the garlic through its unbroken skin as I entered the house. The aroma was so powerful; its pungent fragrance filled the kitchen air. Compare that to a store bought garlic clove and you will find there is no comparison in aroma.

If you ever had the pleasure and good fortune of eating a "Jersey hot-house tomato" from fifty years ago, you may recall its fantastic flavor and color. They were a huge multi-lobed fruit and had a deep, sometimes-purplish red color and a very distinctive tomato flavor. Compare that to a typical store-bought tomato today which is a virtually flavorless, odorless, and lightly colored poor imitation of a tomato. Spinach that was grown in those days had *fifty times* the iron content compared with most spinach grown today. The same is true with virtually all commercially available foods. Compare whole rye bread with its deep color, heavy weight and rich distinctive flavor to *"white bread"* containing chlorinated or brominated bleached flour with its air pockets, a few synthetic vitamins, *"partially hydrogenated oils,"* other artificial ingredients, sugar and preservatives. It has little fiber, minerals, or protein; just *empty calories* that quickly turn to sugar putting a stress on the pancreas and leading to elevated LDL, VLDL (the "bad" cholesterol), triglycerides, weight gain, digestive tract disorders, diabetes, and heart disease. The partially hydrogenated oil alone is one of the leading causes of dietary induced heart disease. One must understand that there are an entire host of *"lethal poisons"* on our grocery shelves adorned with attractive wrappings. These poisons cannot be removed from the marketplace due in large to the modern day need for *"shelf life."* Unfortunately, if you do not avoid these items, increased shelf life in the long run yields decreased human life.

Food processing with the addition of preservatives, sugar, salt, artificial colors, sweeteners, free flowing agents, and flavorings add to the toxic burden and nutritional destruction of our food supply. Furthermore, most people eat a less varied diet consisting of a short list of their "favorite foods." The most commonly consumed *"vegetable"* today is French fries, which are full of hydrogenated oils and rancid fats. Commercially prepared fried foods are cooked in hydrogenated oils and fats that contain toxic preservatives such as BHT and BHA. Due to the high heat and length of time that these commercial oils are used, they are oxidized into toxic by-products. These toxic, rancidified oils and fats have been implicated in increasing the risk of heart disease and cancer. They are pro-inflammatory. Elevated levels of cholesterol, insulin, and triglycerides are widely considered to be cardiovascular risk factors.

The Aloe polymannans and numerous phytonutrients have been shown to lower total cholesterol and triglycerides, reduce elevated insulin, and blood glucose levels; lowering risk factors for cardiovascular disease, obesity, and diabetes. Elevated insulin levels are a factor in obesity because the increased levels of insulin force blood sugar more rapidly into the cells which then must convert it to triglycerides for storage (in fat cells) because it cannot be utilized that rapidly for energy.

The Aloe polysaccharides and numerous phytonutrients also contain antioxidant and anti-inflammatory properties, all of which have protective effects against cardiovascular disease. Due to the fact that 80% of diabetics die from cardiovascular disease, the consumption of these healing components is of particular importance to anyone who has been diagnosed with diabetes.

Overeating Yet Under-Feeding

Many Americans are experiencing difficulty maintaining their desired weight. There are two main reasons for this.

The diet is lacking in essential nutrients which act as catalysts or co-enzymes designed to facilitate metabolism. Without these catalysts, metabolism slows, fewer calories are burned, and more fat is stored. Simply reducing caloric intake does not solve the problem because this further slows the metabolism and also causes weakness and fatigue, promoting inactivity.

The other reason for unwanted fat storage is overeating. Our appetites are over-stimulated and we feel that we are hungry even though we are consuming adequate amounts of food. In most cases, this paradox is due to the fact that the consumption of nutrient poor foods leaves the body hungry because it is starved for the essential nutrients needed to function optimally. Nutrient deprived cells are signaling the body with specific requests required for the performance of their various functions or the production of new cells. This signaling for nutrients continues regardless of the level of caloric intake. Inevitably, fat storage occurs as a result of overeating.

Thus, individuals possessing poor eating habits may consume large quantities of nutrient deficient, high calorie, poor quality foods and yet remain with additional food cravings due to cells crying out for vital missing nutrients. The cells remain under-fed and signaling for quality support. Unfortunately, given the poor quality of most foods available currently, this type of craving-related overeating cycle is a common condition. With nutrient deficient food sources on every corner, it is easy to understand why two out of three Americans are overweight.

Pregnant women experience powerful cravings. These signals originate from cells demanding nutrients for the production of new cells within the developing embryo. This is an obvious example of our innate cellular signaling mechanisms.

Fad diets designed to reduce caloric intake do not work in the long run because they do not address the nutrient deficiency of the cells. Exercise regimes designed to burn calories fail as well for the same reason and simultaneously create a higher demand for quality cellular support. The food cravings and excessive appetite continue unabated while fatigue increases. This fuel-poor, stress-rich cellular environment is an open invitation for disease. Appetite suppressing drugs, often containing dangerous stimulants, only further exacerbate the problem by further depletion of essential nutrients. This explains why most "diets," even if temporarily effective, fail in the long run. THEY DO NOT CORRECT THE UNDERLYING CAUSE OF OBESITY: NUTRIENT DEFICIENCY! The three most common weight loss approaches; calorie restriction, exercise, and the consumption of stimulants or diet drugs all increase the demand for vital nutrients. These approaches utilized without adequate cellular support all become a vicious self-defeating cycle.

Fortunately, the healthy solution for the stabilization of appetite and subsequently the elimination of excess fat storage is to simply provide the body, and subsequently the cells, what they require to operate as designed.

Aloe components and numerous phytonutrients have been shown to stabilize blood sugar levels reducing food cravings. These in conjunction with full spectrum essential minerals support metabolism and are essential for health. They are catalysts or co-enzymes which are required for optimum metabolism. When taken in proper proportions and amounts, healthy metabolism can be achieved over time while nourishing the cells simultaneously. In addition, the spectrum of components we are discussing also work synergistically and are essential for healthy thyroid function. Components from the aloe as well as iodine from the organically bound minerals are also necessary for the production of thyroid hormone.

Many speak joyfully of a spa day, indulging in massage, nail maintenance, and various modes of after-the-fact superficial relief. Would it not be preferable, and vastly more intelligent, to live *a life-long spa day,* rewarding ourselves around the clock from the inside out? The most important thing to remember is that it is never too late to start. Let us love ourselves first, by loving *our cells* first! It is not *selfish;* it is intelligent, and mandatory for quality life.

Essential Co-Factors

The reader may be aware that we, the authors, are continually discussing subjects that the medical establishment and drug cartel do not want the public to understand. The Cartel does not want you to gain the knowledge that the answers to these life-threatening issues are in the least bit understandable and solvable through safe and natural means.

Vitamins and minerals are essential co-factors required for health and even survival. They facilitate metabolism, growth, and repair. They are not optional. There is a long list of nutritional deficiency diseases. Examples are scurvy from lack of vitamin C, Beriberi from lack of B vitamins, rickets from lack of vitamin D, poor night vision from lack of vitamin A, lutein, and xanthene (plant pigments), iron deficiency anemia from lack of iron and pernicious anemia from lack of vitamin B-12 and folic acid. There is even a copper deficiency anemia. Goiter, an abnormal enlargement of the thyroid gland, is caused by a lack of iodine. These are just a few of those deficiency diseases discovered. Zinc and selenium are essential for a healthy prostate gland and immune function. Chromium, vanadium, zinc, and magnesium are needed for the maintenance of normal blood sugar levels; beta phytosterol (found in Aloe vera) has been very helpful in eliminating benign prostatic hypertrophy. Selenium (also found in Aloe) aids the function of vitamin E, also in aloe, and has been associated with reduced rates of cancer. There are of course many more examples which could be given. Multitudes are suffering to varying degrees with these and many other diseases and disorders without being *"officially diagnosed."*

C.I.C.D.S. (Cellular and Immune Communication Deficiency Syndrome) will prove not only to be the most overlooked deficiency disease, but in the future will be recognized of fundamental importance involving the majority of degenerative diseases presently known to man. Due to its foundational and widespread nature, and subsequently its involvement in so many different disease processes, we have termed it a syndrome, rather than a single disease.

With the replacement of these essential carbohydrate and organically bound nutrients, we have witnessed the normalization of blood sugar levels, the elimination of food cravings and excessive weight, the elimination of gastric ulcers, severe ulcerative colitis, diarrhea, irritable bowel syndrome, and other gastrointestinal diseases, the increase of killer T cells (reversal of immune suppression), improvement in the health of skin (including elimination of abnormal skin growths and the elimination of psoriasis, eczema, dermatitis, and rosacea) as well as numerous other health conditions.

Biochemical texts and scientific literature including research articles from around the world all point to the enormous need to bring this nutritional deficiency syndrome to light. By correcting this virtually universal nutritional deficiency there will be a vast improvement in the health of innumerable people throughout the world. The ingestion of these polysaccharides and organically bound phytonutrients on a regular basis will act to prevent, reduce the frequency, and heal widespread degenerative diseases.

As more researchers and physicians utilize these essential carbohydrate and organically bound nutrients, many more therapeutic uses will inevitably arise. As discussed throughout this book; The cure, and preferably the prevention of the majority of degenerative diseases and conditions known to man, is the daily ingestion of a comprehensive, full spectrum of disease- fighting, immune-boosting, bioactive phytonutrients in adequate amounts. In addition, we must avoid the obvious pitfalls of health, the poisons within many foods, drinks, and substances currently on the market.

The *SLOW* DEATH LIST

Avoid all of the following as much as possible:

Hydrogenated and partially hydrogenated oils, "trans" fats, and other poor quality oils: Poor quality oils added to processed foods include cottonseed, peanut, canola, and soybean oils. For several reasons including the fact that they have poor omega III to omega VI ratios and may contain pesticides and harmful solvents, they should be avoided. Fats and oils which have positive health benefits include: Extra virgin olive oil, grapeseed oil (high antioxidant content and raises HDL), coconut oil (resists oxidation, promotes weight loss). Organic butter or coconut oil is excellent for sautéing and baking.

Cigarettes: The only product that is legally sold that kills an estimated one third of its customers. Tobacco products contain one of the most addictive substances known; nicotine. They also contain high levels of radioactive compounds and heavy metals such as cadmium (carcinogenic) and numerous toxic by-products. It has been estimated that one puff of a cigarette contains billions of free radicals, increasing the need for antioxidant or free radical scavengers.

Caffeine: A large segment of the public is *"addicted"* to caffeine, and in particular, coffee. The harmful effects of caffeine on the human body could fill this book. Many rely on coffee or other forms of caffeine to "wake up" or for *"energy"* in general. Lack of energy is due to poor cellular nutrition and health habits in general.

Soda: Carbonated drinks such as colas, and others, are highly acidic. They often contain phosphoric acid, carbonic acid, sugar or artificial sweeteners, caffeine, artificial colors, brominated oil, and other chemical additives. The high acidity and sugar content causes the parathyroid glands to secrete elevated levels of parathormone. This forces the bones to release calcium into the blood, thereby causing osteoporosis and dental cavities. They have a negative nutritive value, containing none of the needed nutrients or phytonutrients so essential for optimum health.

Pharmaceuticals: If the drug or pharmaceutical is synthetic *(and 99% are)* and/or produces *"side effects"* (and most do), which we know are direct unwanted harmful effects, marketed *"to the side"* for less *negative* curb appeal, be sure that these are eroding your cells and thus your health with varying degrees of speed and severity. Unfortunately, many drugs cannot be suddenly abandoned without potential adverse reactions. **Note:** See Your Licensed "Health Care" Practitioner Before Discontinuing Any Medications.

Hard liquor: Hard liquor has empty calories and no nutritionally redeeming qualities. Alcohol increases the risks of many degenerative diseases. The bodies' natural processes to detoxify itself from the alcohol are a nutritional drain on the body as well.

Sugar and artificial sweeteners: The only sweetener we recommend is natural stevia. Increased sugar consumption has been implicated in diabetes, hyperactivity, and obesity. The addition of *refined* sugars, particularly table sugar (sucrose) and fructose (refined from fruit) should be avoided as much as possible. Clarification; Do not avoid fruit; avoid fructose refined *from* fruit due to the high concentrations.

Artificial colors and flavors: These synthetic agents have no nutritive value, are often used to cover-up nutritional deficiencies and have been repeatedly shown to cause health problems.

Preservatives: Avoid food preservatives as much as possible. Nitrates and nitrites, for example, have been implicated as a causative agent in colon cancer. Many preservatives are anti-enzymes and therefore inhibit digestion and metabolism.

Municipal or tap water: Avoid municipal or tap waters as they have been found to contain chlorine, fluorine, organic wastes, other chemicals and harmful substances. Drink spring water, mineral water, or use a filtration system.

Food Recommendations for Optimum Health

Beauty Without Substance

Fruits and Vegetables:

While standing in the supermarket holding a large, plump, red tomato in our hands, it is hard to imagine that this beautiful piece of fruit may be void of the essential nutrients for which it was designed to deliver. In fact, size and color of produce has no bearing on nutritional content. Commercial farmers need to yield high crop volumes to turn a profit and survive. In order for the planted crop to yield high volumes of produce, today's nutrient depleted soils must be fertilized. Most often if not always with commercial farming, artificial fertilizers are used which supply the plant with nutrients it needs to produce *larger volumes*. While creating larger plants, higher yields, and *"beautiful"* produce, the grave dilemma is that these artificial fertilizers do not provide the soil, and subsequently the plant, with many minerals which are vital to *the human*. Furthermore, artificial fertilizers, herbicides, and pesticides suppress vital soil micro-organisms thus diminishing the "life" of the soil and hindering the many complex and often poorly understood biological processes needed for nutrient supply to the plants. The combined result is large, pretty and plentiful produce, void of specific and significant vital human phytonutrient content.

"Certified Organic"

"Certified Organic" soil standards are designed to protect and encourage soil micro-organisms which are necessary to *unlock* nutrients from the soil. The conversion period of three years is required before a farm is awarded *"full organic status."* This requirement, in part, is to allow the soil's microbiological life to recover and multiply.

Nevertheless, *"Certified Organic"* is **not** an assurance of significant quantities of phytonutrients. "Certified Organic" is a designation indicating that the certified food is free from synthetic chemicals such as artificial fertilizers and pesticides, and that the farmland (soil) has been free of these contaminants for three years or more.

Although we recommend *"Certified Organic"* fruits and vegetables be consumed as much as possible, we need to make this distinction clear that the organic certification *is **not** a guarantee* of nutrient content as well. Because there is no requirement that the soil be enriched with organic fertilizer, too often *"organically certified"* fruits and vegetables are being grown in nutrition-depleted soils, just as commercial produce is. To enrich the soil naturally after decades of abuse, neglect and depletion, it will take many years of diligent application of intensive organic farming techniques. Unfortunately, this is generally not commercially viable.

Additionally, whether commercially grown or organic, most fruits and vegetables delivered to market today are harvested green before they completely ripened on the plant. This is done to avoid loss due to spoilage in transit and on the shelf. This **"green-harvesting"** robs the plant of the opportunity to deliver a significant portion of the phytonutrients to the produce in the critical last 3-5 days of ripening.

As if all this were not enough, cooking foods also destroys many phytonutrients. Molecular changes take place in nutrients as foods are cooked above 115 degrees Fahrenheit for just a few minutes. Damage progressively worsens at higher temperatures over longer periods of time. The degree of nutrient destruction is simply a matter of temperature, cooking method, and time. Microwave ovens are said to destroy up to 90% of the nutrient content within foods. (Vegetables should be steamed for one to three minutes depending on thickness or stir-fried in healthy oils such as olive, grapeseed, coconut, or clarified organic butter, and served immediately).

The industrial revolution, commencing in the early 19th century, has progressively contaminated our environment, and subsequently our bodies. In this age of increasing toxic pollutants, the amount of anti-oxidants our cells require to eliminate free radicals and prevent cellular damage has quite conceivably risen dramatically from just a few generations ago. While the need has risen, the supply has simultaneously fallen for many of the same reasons listed. As a result, we are receiving a mere fraction of the phytonutrient/ anti-oxidant protection and regenerative bio-chemical fuel we require for optimum health.

This makes the consumption of higher volumes of raw fruits and properly cooked or raw vegetables in conjunction with phytonutrient-rich supplementation critical. Despite having a varied diet including a wide variety of organic foods, it is virtually impossible to obtain adequate amounts of phytonutrients from the modern food supply alone. In addition, specific vital phytonutrients are missing from the food supply altogether. Nevertheless, in regard to fruits and vegetables, "certified organic" is preferable.

Meats and Poultry:

Due to the fact that pesticides are concentrated in the fatty tissues of animals, and hormones and antibiotics are frequently used in commercially raised meats, we recommend the consumption of "natural," "organic," or "free range" meats and poultry. Organically raised eggs are preferable for the very same reasons.

Seafood:

We recommend the consumption of "wild caught" fish and shellfish. Avoid *"farm raised"* varieties. These are fed an antibiotic laden, unnatural diet of corn meal. They are also fed coloring agents to visually substitute for the natural color of the wild variety that is not present in farm raised due to the absence of the natural nutrient-rich diet of wild fish.

Breads and Grains:

Consume whole grain sprouted natural breads. The process of *sprouting* generates many important phytonutrients. Avoid breads made from bleached or brominated flours (white breads). These also often contain partially hydrogenated oils, sugar, and preservatives with a few synthetic vitamins added. They have little fiber and virtually no nutritional benefit. Whole grains such as brown rice, wild rice, millet, buckwheat, whole steel cut oats and quinoa are examples of nutrient rich grains. There are many whole grains available today. They are far superior nutritionally compared to refined and processed grains.

Dairy Products:

We only recommend dairy products which are certified organic. Commercial dairy production in the U.S. is rampant with antibiotics, synthetic bovine hormones, and grain feeding rather than grass. Grain feeding lowers the omega III content. Certified organic dairy products, especially "high vitamin butter" derived from cows that are grazed on rapidly growing grass, is an excellent source of vitamins A and D and omega III essential fatty acids. Dairy products such as milk, cheese, and yogurt are high in calcium. Cultured organic dairy products such as yogurt and kefir are superior as they are already partially pre-digested, have lower lactose content, and contain "friendly bacteria." Organic cheese contains "high density nutrition." In contrast, "American cheese" is of poor quality and has additives such as vegetable oil. Sanitation can be a problem in *"factory farms"* where the cattle are not permitted to "free range" and graze on grass, their natural diet.

Nutritional Supplements:

If the nutritional supplement is synthetic or inorganic, avoid it. Although it is difficult to obtain the majority of nutritional supplements in a natural organic form, choose these vitamins, minerals, and phytonutrients from natural organic sources as much as possible.

Beverages:

Water is best (see below). Herbal teas such as chamomile and green tea are very good in general. Organic rice milk is very easy to digest and is great for mixing supplements. Unsweetened 100% natural fruit and vegetable juices are excellent. An occasional beer or glass of red wine is not harmful. Beer, including the non-alcoholic variety, is made with purified water and contains B vitamins. Red wine contains Resveratrol and proanthocyanidans; powerful antioxidants. Organic wine will not contain sulfites or pesticide residues and is preferable. With alcoholic beverages, moderation is obviously the key!

Note: Adequate water consumption is at least partially determined by activity level and how much one perspires. We recommend six - eight ounce glasses of water for a sedentary person, and eight to ten - eight ounce glasses of water or more for the more active. Thirst alone is not the best indicator of the need for water. Generally, the bulk of needed water intake is best consumed between meals so as to not dilute your digestive juices, slowing digestion and reducing absorption of nutrients. Water is partially responsible for literally every metabolic process in the human body. Water is the largest single constituent of the body and is essential for cellular homeostasis. Intracellular water (fluids inside the cells) accounts for approximately 65% of our total body water and extracellular water (water around the cells) about 35%. The intracellular-extracellular water exchange transports nutrients to needed areas and aids in the removal of toxins from the cells. Adequate hydration is a key factor of health. Cell dehydration can often lead to oxygen starvation, premature-aging, and an entire host of diseases.

"Food pyramids" are both hopeless and impossible guidelines

The 2005 USDA dietary guidelines recommend 9 servings of fruits and vegetables daily. The National Cancer Society admits that the former "5-a-day" gospel was just the "bare minimum." Nonetheless, it is routinely reported that only 1 in 5 adults follow this flawed advice to any consistent degree and even less children do.

The reasons their number of recommended daily servings are continually rising is twofold. First there is the perpetuating volume of research showing phytonutrients to be the answer. Second is the scientific data confirming the stark declines in nutrient content of modern produce. The phytonutrient content within most fruits and vegetables grown today is miserably low.

Due to this vastly deficient phytonutrient content, even the current recommendations of 9 servings daily are grossly inadequate from a potency perspective, especially for an individual currently suffering from disease. Nevertheless, how could they possibly recommend more when the current recommendations are close to impossible to follow? A person would need to spend the better part of the day chewing, barely able to leave the table.

Once again, herein lies the problem. As a result of this produce nutrient deficiency, the public serving recommendation to acquire sufficient phytonutrient intake for optimum health, in reality, may be as many as 50 daily servings of fruits and vegetables.

Unfortunately, if the government provides the real unreachable daily serving figure to the public, it would be discouraging to those attempting to consume, and embarrassing to those reporting. True disclosure would also expose the national food crisis which would be disadvantageous to corporate America. Disclosing the true necessary serving figures for optimum health would also place too much of an emphasis on the need for phytonutrients as the answer to **The Plague,** and starkly erode the manufactured public faith in the medical-drug-based "healthcare" system.

Most people consume a relatively narrow range of foods which *they like,* certain meats, certain carbohydrates, certain fruits and vegetables at best. In addition, they consume harmful products such as soda, bleached flour, refined sugar, additives, preservatives etc. Most of these food sources are lacking vital nutrients. They may take a few synthetic vitamins in the belief that this will make up for the lack in their diets, but this is a fantasy and the current rates of degenerative disease lend stark confirmation to this.

Phytonutrient Supplementation

With all factors considered, the vital phytonutrients contained in one serving of fruits or vegetables 100 years ago may be for the sake of argument, the equivalent of approximately 10 servings of fruits or vegetables today. With most Americans finding the ingestion of 50 or more daily servings impossible, phytonutrient supplementation is more than "a good idea," it is no less than **critical.** We are all suffering from cellular starvation, from the continual lack of specific and sufficient phytonutrient intake.

Furthermore, combined with the cost and impracticality of consuming 9-30 daily servings of fruits and vegetables in an attempt to acquire adequate phytonutrient intake, the practice would be undesirable from a caloric standpoint.

A strong scientific argument for phytonutrient supplementation in today's nutrient poor food environment is the science of *caloric restriction.* Caloric restriction is a well documented anti-aging strategy. Numerous studies have shown that the practice of restricting calorie intake while maintaining diverse nutritional status improves multiple aspects of age-related decline. Caloric restriction involves the elimination of nutrient-poor foods containing empty calories replaced by nutrient-dense foods and supplementation. Caloric restriction accomplishes this by producing changes in gene expression that are associated with long life and a slowing of the aging process.

Take Your Cod Liver Oil!

Cod liver oil once highly recommended, has fallen from popularity due in part to its strong taste and smell. Fortunately, today, flavored cod liver oil allows us to benefit from this super supplement without the fishy taste.

The health benefits of cod liver oil are numerous and synergistic. Cod liver oil has been shown to be important for the development of the nervous system. It is thought to be of benefit in preventing learning disabilities. High levels of the elongated Omega III fats EPA and DHA, essential for prostaglandin (regulatory hormones) and brain development are present. It is a neurological wonder which improves brain function, stress response, memory, learning disorders, bipolar syndrome and manic-depression. It is also effective in improving immune response and alleviating allergies and asthma. It protects against childhood leukemia and lung cancer, prevents rickets in the young and osteoporosis in the elderly. It is effective in treating arthritis. It reduces inflammation, helps relax blood vessels, and reduces pain and damage in inflamed joints. Patients of all ages with colitis respond more favorably to cod liver oil than medication.

Cod liver oil contains vitamins A, D and K which support immune function, calcium absorption, and blood clotting. Alternative treatments for cancer have emphasized *natural* vitamin A. Cod liver oil lowers blood pressure from elevated cortisol levels. It promotes absorption of calcium and magnesium, thereby lowering blood pressure which helps protect against glaucoma. It has been documented to reduce morbidity and mortality in children. Pregnant women taking cod liver oil have infants with lower risk of Type 1 diabetes. Cod liver oil has been shown to improve glucose response in adult diabetics with both Type 1 and Type 2 diabetes.

According to Weston Price, DDS, who conducted a worldwide anthropological study, the consumption of "high vitamin butter" along with the "high vitamin cod liver oil" produced the best effects. This is likely due to the fact that the essential fatty acids in cod liver oil are better utilized and stored in the presence of saturated fats. A word about "saturated fats" and cholesterol; Saturated fats and cholesterol are essential for health and life itself. All membranes in your body contain cholesterol. It is the building block of all hormones. We do not want *oxidized* or *rancidified* fats and oils, nor do we want elevated LDL, VLDL, triglycerides or low HDL, or other markers of cardiovascular disease. Whenever considering cholesterol levels, the higher the HDL, the higher the safe level of total cholesterol.

Despite the long term use and immense amount of positive research regarding cod liver oil, and the fact that *low* vitamin A *causes birth defects,* it is no longer recommended in the U.S. or Great Britain for use by pregnant women! This is so because of a non-specific and therefore misleading report of November 23, 1995, published in the New England Journal of Medicine which showed birth defects with intake of mostly *synthetic* vitamin A exceeding 5000iu daily. Once again, the *Synthetic* form being the culprit. *Accutane*, another *synthetic* vitamin A, has also been shown to be associated with birth defects. There is a recognized teratogenicity (causes birth defects) of retinoic acid, a *synthetic form* of vitamin A. This is yet another example of why we stress the natural organic form of nutrients rather than synthetic ones.

Levels up to 30,000iu of preformed vitamin A (from natural sources), are considered safe. 30,000iu is the equivalent of 12 teaspoons, more than anyone would likely take. High levels of vitamin A may be dangerous in persons with liver disease such as alcoholic cirrhosis. Imported cod liver oil is tested for contaminants. Mercury compounds are water soluble so they do not contaminate it.

Nutritional Protocol for Prevention, Anti-Aging, and Disease Recovery

As a general guideline; Optimum Health may be achieved by:

1. Reasonable *Avoidance* of the **SLOW DEATH LIST**, as much as, and whenever possible. (This is necessary to avoid cellular damage in general).

2. The daily maintenance of the digestive tract and immune system, the doorway to health, disease prevention, and recovery. (Ingest the immune modulating components pages 60-62) (AUTOIMMUNE-X)

3. Eating and drinking ***sufficient amounts** of the recommended foods and beverages above.

4. Supplementation with phytonutrients whenever possible.

5. The daily ingestion of one to two tablespoons of cod liver oil.

6. Daily moderate sunshine and fresh air. **If possible: In the early morning or late afternoon, when the sun non-direct and better filtered by the atmosphere,** receive up to one hour sunshine per day, preferably in an area where fresh air is prevalent and noise a minimum. (adjust the time exposure to better suit your skin-type). This is necessary to receive adequate amounts of critical vitamin D, and other benefits from the sun. (*See pages 115)

7. Sufficient exercise tailored to your age and individual physical condition.

*Sufficient caloric intake and hydration amounts vary for each individual based on sex, age, weight, muscle-mass, daily activity levels, and possibly genetic factors. Note: Individual results may vary. This optimum health guideline is based primarily on nutrition. Other factors of optimum health may also apply, such as daily exercise and stress reduction techniques. Other natural supplements may be advisable for specific existing conditions. See your licensed healthcare practitioner prior to commencing an exercise regime and for all medical advice.

The Common Fruits and Vegetables List

Although there are hundreds of fruits and vegetables grown throughout the world, the following is a list of the more common, easily accessible ones:

Common Fruits:

Acai, Apples, Apricot, Avocados, Black mulberries, Blackberries, Blueberries, Cherries, Coconut, Cranberries, Elderberries, Gooseberries, Grapefruit, Grapes, Guava, Huckleberries, Jujube Key Lime, Kiwifruit, Kumquat, Lemons, Limes, Loquat, Lychee, Nectarines, Olives, Oranges, Papaya, Peaches, Pear, Pineapple, Plums, Pomegranates, Prunes, Raisins, Raspberries, Strawberries, Tangerines, Tomatoes, Watermelon, Wolfberries

Common Vegetables:

Artichoke, Arugula, Asparagus, Beans, Beet, Broccoli, Broccoli, Rabe, Brussel Sprouts, Cabbage, Carrot, Cauliflower, Cilantro, Celery, Chard, Collard greens, Corn, Cucumber, Dandelion greens, Kale, Kohlrabi, Leek, Lettuce, Okra, Onions, Parsley, Parsnips Peppers, Potatoes, Pumpkin, Radishes, Rhubarb, Rutabagas, Shallots, Spinach, Squash, Sweet potato, Tomatoes, Turnips, Watercress, Yams

Here Comes the Sun

One of the current establishment's favorite *"look out for nature warnings,"* is their effort to label the sun and exposure to the sun as sinister. Let us examine this *brilliant* concept for a moment. The sun is the center of the universe. All that is known within our universe revolves around the sun. The sun is the source of life for every living organism on the planet. In plants, the sun generates *photosynthesis,* in turn creating oxygen and the entire food supply for all living creatures. In humans, direct sunlight on the skin produces Vitamin D. Photosynthetically produced vitamin D facilitates the absorption of calcium, a master nutrient critical for life and other critical nutrients in the small intestine. Simultaneously, photosynthesis also results in the production of inositol triphosphate, INSP-3, a calcium chelator, which serves to regulate extraction of calcium stored in the cells. Sunshine on the skin and subsequently the production of Vitamin D increases mineral absorption, thereby reducing acidosis known to promote degenerative diseases including cancer. Cancer rates in the regions closer to the equator where sunshine is more prevalent and intense are a fraction of the incidence of cancer in the northern regions farther away.

Indirect sunlight entering the eyes influences the pituitary and pineal glands, the master glands which control the entire endocrine system. Sunlight is a nutrient essential to life and the secretion of hormones. In all, greater availability to unfiltered sunlight is of great health benefit if, like anything else of value, received in intelligent moderation.

For the most part, modern man dwells in an indoor world comprised of artificial lighting. The amount of sunlight he receives through his modern attire is but a fraction of the sunlight enjoyed by his predecessors. The current plague of degenerative diseases also appears to be in line with man's urban and suburban indoor retreat.

Here is a short list of diseases related to *lack of* sunlight; breast cancer, colon cancer, diabetes, elevated blood pressure, heart disease, multiple sclerosis, ovarian cancer, osteomalacia, osteoporosis, prostate cancer, psoriasis, rickets, seasonal affective disorder, tooth decay, and tuberculosis.

*Not only is sunshine "good for you," sunshine is excellent and critical for your overall health. Numerous studies have been conducted involving those whom, for extended periods, work by night and sleep during the day receiving little if any sunlight. The overall state of health of night dwellers in comparison to children of the light is in short, *night and day*. Again, as with most things in life, moderation and individualized precautions are key. Unless you have skin cancer, the *dim-witted* advice proclaiming *"stay out of the sun,"* is not only vague and irresponsible, but scientifically ignorant.

Studies have confirmed that the higher the latitude in which you live, (less sun) the more likely you are to die of cancer.

Journal of the National Cancer Institute (JNCI): *"increased* sun *exposure reduces the risk of non-Hodgkin's lymphoma." (cancer)*

That said: increased sun *reduces risk of* cancer.

(JNCI): *"evidence is beginning to emerge that sunlight exposure, particularly as it relates to the vitamin D synthesized in the skin under the influence of solar radiation, might have a beneficial influence for certain cancers."*

The health risks associated with receiving *inadequate* amounts of vitamin D (i.e. sun exposure) involve not only cancer, but an entire host of degenerative diseases.

Once again, it would seem that the establishment is advising us to avoid the natural component that provides the prevention and cure by design, SENDING US IN THE EXACT OPPOSITE DIRECTION – THE DIRECTION OF DISEASE. Consistently, in almost every area we examine, we can see that The Establishment's misinformation will slowly harm, if not eventually kill us.☺

*See recommendations page 119 for tips on intelligent sunlight ex- posure. Those individuals considered a high risk may require protection practices and should subsequently confer with their medical practitioner to establish a balance between sun exposure and food or supplementation to obtain adequate amounts of vital Vitamin D.

Chapter 5

The Current
State of
"Modern Medicine"

Schizo-Care U.S.A.

Diseases are out of control in America, and to a great extent in most industrial countries today due to a schizophrenic (insane split-personality) approach to healthcare that has been proclaimed as mainstream. On the one hand, in America, we have the largest most technologically advanced and most expensive system of healthcare existing anywhere in the world. Currently the U.S. annual healthcare bill is two trillion dollars, and yet *The World Health Organization* ranks the U.S. at *Thirty-Seventh* in health. What an incredibly disgraceful report card! Fifty percent (50%) of the U.S. population will die from cardiovascular disease, forty-two percent (42%) of Americans will be diagnosed at some time with cancer; 24% will die from it. There are 20 million diabetics in America; ONE SIXTH OF THE TOTAL WORLD NUMBER OF 120 MILLION, yet, we are only 5% of the world population. Therefore, Americans are three and one-third times as likely to develop diabetes compared to other citizens of the world. Sixty percent (60%) or more of Americans are overweight. Infections are the third most common cause of death, adverse drug reactions are the fourth. Fifty percent (50%) of all medical diagnosis are incorrect. Drug reactions kill 100,000 patients per year. In 1995, there were 10.8 million visits for the "adverse effects of medical treatments."

"The problems that exist in the world today cannot be solved by the level of thinking that created them." Albert Einstein

Unfortunately, this *"high-tech"* approach is not working. Extraordinarily expensive hospitals, diagnostic equipment, "research facilities," over-prescribed dangerous and abused drugs as well as stressed out personnel are not raising the pitiful standard of health in this country.

Other than crisis intervention, **Symptom Relief Roulette** is the only game they are offering. In regard to the treatment of disease, this system employs a symptomatic approach using drugs that rarely if ever, provide a *cure* for anything. They generally treat symptoms only, creating adverse *side-effects* (which in truth are direct unwanted effects), contraindications (specific high-risk usage), and toxicity. An approach centered on the treatment of symptoms without addressing root-causes of disease is arguably the prolonging of or *"maintenance"* of disease. This structure is clearly *"disease care"* not health care. This system is not structured to provide true health care, but rather it is structured as *a business with disease* where the on-going disease continues to generate revenue.

Treatments such as chemotherapy and radiation are for the most part either ineffectual or temporary. They are generally extremely dangerous, expensive, and often wind up destroying the quality of life of the patient as well as often contributing to their eventual demise. Cure rates for most cancer treatments have improved little over many years and cancer rates are up. It is estimated that one in eight women living in the U.S. will be diagnosed with breast cancer.

Many psychotropic drugs prescribed for psychiatric diagnoses such as: depression, bi-polar, manic, manic depression, schizophrenia, etc., are designed to elevate neurotransmitters such as serotonin. Although serotonin is a necessary neurotransmitter for normal brain function, elevated levels are not beneficial. Serotonergic agents are those that elevate serotonin levels or disrupt its breakdown and have a long list of terrible side-effects including, but not limited to: diabetes, weight gain, irritability, depression, suicidal thoughts, and violence. The Establishment seems to be creating the very diseases they are supposedly treating.

The list of diseases in which serotonin is elevated includes: schizophrenia, mongoloidism, and Alzheimer's. Other psychiatric drugs produce Tardive Dyskinesia which produces wild, dyscoordinated gesticulations, drooling, and permanent neurological damage. What does the PDR (Physicians Desk Reference) say to do in many instances? INCREASE THE DOSE!

Non-steroidal anti-inflammatory drugs (NSAIDS) such as ibuprophen and acetaminophen actually suppress the chondrocytes' (cells that make cartilage) ability to produce cartilage, thereby worsening arthritis. **Actually, most drugs, if taken long enough, will cause or worsen the actual condition for which they had originally been prescribed.** Another example is diuretics, commonly prescribed for high blood pressure and congestive heart failure, cause the kidneys to excrete more fluid. Unfortunately, long-term diuretic use causes kidney damage, thereby putting more stress on the heart and often raising blood pressure or contributing to congestive heart failure.

Statins (cholesterol lowering medications) interfere with the production of essential Co enzyme Q-10, necessary for muscular function (particularly the heart). Despite the fact that these drugs have not been determined to increase life expectancy and that approximately 30% of the patients taking them will experience muscle weakness or other associated musculoskeletal problems, they continue to be prescribed. Again, quite often *"the answer"* is to simply increase the dose of the drug which of course will soon worsen the problem. Another example is the use of Haldol, a psychiatric medication that causes Tardive Dyskinesia (uncontrollable discoordinated movements). What is the protocol (according to The Physicians Desk Reference")? Once again, INCREASE THE DOSE!

Through the mastery of marketing The Cartel persists in the creation of an image portraying themselves as being *"in search of"* the causes and the cures for countless diseases. Expendable as we appear to be, they seem to have created the perception that pharmaceuticals are the answers to the woes of health, and that those who are dying in ever increasing numbers from the ravages of degenerative disease are *"dying in the fight to find the answers."* Although medicine is winning a few highly publicized battles, it is rapidly losing the war on degenerative disease because the only answer that is acceptable to the establishment is a patentable drug.

Many of us have been conditioned from birth to believe that government and big business have our interests at heart. We Americans live in the *"Greatest Country in the World,"* so we are told, and it feels good to believe that we are safe and looked after by our system. It feels good to believe that integrity remains strong in our culture, especially when it comes to the care of the health of our citizens, young and old.

The reality is that integrity **does** reign supreme in the hearts of the majority of those involved in the health care system. Unfortunately, those at the bottom and middle rungs of the ladder, including our doctors, do not make the policies governing the dissemination of vital information which determines the quality of our lives. Most doctors within the system are well intentioned, yet simply unaware of the magnitude of deception and censorship from above.

Drugs Gone Wild!

The following examples are provided to illustrate *the lunacy* of the products and protocols being marketed or *strong-armed* to us in the name of *"modern health care"* and well-being. We use the term strong- armed due to the fact that many patients have been threatened dismissal from their doctors' *"care,"* should they not agree with or fail to follow the drug protocol as recommended. In addition, due to the relentless bombardment of pharmaceutical ads and the medical community's support of most drugs being *approved,* it is very difficult for the patient to consciously withstand *"the system,"* short of resigning from the system entirely.

In regard to the lunacy, for example, statins, widely used cardiovascular (heart) pharmaceuticals will lower cholesterol levels but have not been proven to add one day to life expectancy. To think about it, why would one attempt to raise or lower the level of any substance within the body while risking numerous side effects that may reduce the quality of life, if that endeavor promises not to yield a single extra day of life? They have numerous side effects such as musculoskeletal pains and weakness. Dr. Bruce West states that statins also reduce the levels of Coenzyme Q-10, A VITAL HEART AND MUSCLE NUTRIENT which is essential to the function of all muscles and to life itself! By the way, the company that produced Lipitor, a commonly prescribed statin, knew this, and even patented a Lipitor/Co Enzyme Q-10 formula that was never released.

The over-prescribing of antibiotics has created *"super bugs"* that are increasingly resistant to treatment. Antibiotics also commonly create secondary diseases such as fungal overgrowth (yeast infections). Furthermore, antibiotics will often indiscriminately destroy the "friendly bacteria" which normally inhabit our lower digestive tract. These bacteria are essential to our health as they are not only the natural enemies of the pathogenic (disease-causing bacteria and fungi), but produce essential B vitamins, break down certain complex carbohydrates for numerous uses, and produce vitamin K essential for blood clotting.

In reality, VIRTUALLY EVERY DRUG, IF TAKEN LONG ENOUGH WILL CAUSE THE VERY DISEASE FOR WHICH IT IS PRESCRIBED, AND AS PROVEN REPEATEDLY, CAUSE OTHER SYMPTOMS AND DISEASES. As mentioned, non-steroidal anti-inflammatory drugs such as those mentioned above destroy the chondrocytes' (cartilage building cells) ability to function and will over time reduce the amount of cartilage your body is able to produce thereby worsening arthritis, leading to further joint destruction!

The side effects, which are actually direct effects of most psychiatric drugs, are psychiatric symptoms such as; depression, confusion, nervousness, restlessness, dizziness, light-headedness, fainting, headache, and insomnia!

AZT, one of the original drugs used to treat HIV infection (AIDS) causes "acquired immune deficiency." Hard to believe? It is clearly stated in the PDR (physicians desk reference). Interestingly, AZT was initially produced as a chemotherapeutic agent to treat cancer, but was taken off the market because it was considered to be too dangerous. It was too immunosuppressive. In other words, its major *"side effect"* was acquired immune deficiency!

Yet another example, if you did not have diabetes and you took insulin, in time your body would make less insulin and you would be, in effect, diabetic! This would occur because the sensors that stimulate the pancreas to release insulin would become *satiated* and would no longer call for the production of more insulin. This is why diabetics become more and more dependent on their insulin. The same is true for patients taking synthetic thyroid medications. These patients are often told that once they start taking these drugs, they will be dependent on them for the rest of their lives. The same is often true of high blood pressure medication such as diuretics, which are known to cause kidney disease (a leading cause of hypertension; high blood pressure). If there is an immunological aspect to any disease, such as Crohn's, ulcerative colitis, rheumatoid arthritis, lupus, MS, etc., taking steroid medications will condemn these patients to life-long problems due to their well-documented immunosuppressive effects.

In January, 1996, an article was published in the Journal of the American Medical Association entitled, *"Carcinogenicity of Cholesterol Lowering Drugs"* by Dr. T.B. Newman and Dr. S. B. Hulley from San Francisco University Medical School. They demonstrated that most of the cholesterol lowering drugs on the market, namely statins and fibrates, cause cancer in test animals taking levels equal to humans. Many of these drugs are still on the market today as cancer rates continue to ravage our society.

By the year 1900, cancer was attacking just 3 out of 100 Americans. By 1950, cancer afflicted 20 out of 100 Americans. In 2017, the NIH stated that approximately 39.5 percent of men and women will be diagnosed with cancer at some point during their lifetime. If we don't change our method of attack, by the end of the century it may afflict virtually everyone.

We have provided only a few examples illustrating how pharmaceutical medications often produce the very opposite effect of what was desired by the patient. This illogical approach, driven by industry profits, literally condemns the patient to a lifetime of the disorder or disease for which they originally sought treatment. This abomination perpetuates *"lifetime clients"* for the industry.

The pharmaceutical industry has no incentive to let these facts be known by the public, and has every incentive to hide them.

Doctor and author, John Abramson – Harvard University, states; *"During the 1990s, most research got pulled out of the universities and was brought to for-profit research organizations. The problem is that gave virtually complete control over the research to the drug companies."*

Jerome Hoffman M.D. - UCLA Medical School, states: *"If we want to be different we have to insist on it. We have to have the clout and the influence and the organization to make it so that they can't blithely go along making the FDA be something that has been widely and famously called a servant of the drug industry. We have to make it so the FDA is a servant of us."*

The presence of Cellular and Immune Communication Deficiency Syndrome (C.I.C.D.S) predisposes us to a wide variety of health problems including chronic degenerative diseases which reduce the quality of human life and longevity.

Decades of the drug-based allopathic medical philosophy, which almost completely ignores prevention through comprehensive cellular nutrition, has brought us into in era of widespread diseases.

They have most of the public *believing* that *"we just **get** these diseases as we get old."*

The Biological Terrain

The cornerstone of *"modern medicine's"* allopathic (the treatment of *disease*) approach is based on French chemist Louis Pasteur's *"germ theory of disease,"* also called the *pathogenic theory of medicine* originating in the mid-1800's.

It is a theory that proposes that microorganisms are <u>the cause</u> of many diseases. Therefore, the microorganism is the main focus, the enemy, and must be eliminated. Once the invader is killed, the body will return to normal. This is the image of *"disease"* the public has been sold for well over a century and a half now.

While scientists rarely dispute that *germs* or *microorganisms* can play an integral role in disease, the fact is that the science of the time, as well as modern science today recognizes that *"the germ theory"* is incomplete and therefore misleading as a theory of disease <u>by itself.</u> It is a fractional truth of reality.

At the time of Louis Pasteur, peer and archrival Antoine Bechamp, MD, PhD, was one of France's most active researchers and cell biologists. Bechamp stated, *"Germs do not cause disease in the real sense. Something happens in the body to allow the germ to become invasive."* In other words, the environment changes favoring the germ and the defense mechanisms of the body fail to overcome and eliminate the invader.

During this same period, Claude Bernard, another French scientist concurring with Bechamp, developed the theory that the host's internal environment was more important in determining disease than the germ. Bernard stated, *"if the internal terrain was an inhospitable place for disease to flourish, then the disease could never overtake the host."* This means that disease usually arises from within the body, that healthy microorganisms always exist within the body, and microorganisms change and transform based on their environment. Microorganisms become dangerous when there are unhealthy conditions within the body.

Ironically upon his death bed, Louis Pasteur openly conceded; *"The germ is nothing, the terrain is everything."* Meaning, the state of health of the body (the environment or terrain) is the main factor determining disease and the presence of *"the germ"* played a fractional role at best.

Any competent scientist understands this today. Nevertheless, the allopathic establishment had already settled on the germ theory to carry its cause and effect philosophy. This incomplete theory (fractional-theory) is *the excuse* harbored by the Pharma/ Medical Establishment which *legitimizes* their allopathic approach to treatment and *justifies* the administering of profitable but harmful drugs and invasive, expensive, and most often unnecessary medical procedures. It is this incomplete theory that allows the establishment to treat the disease, *"the germ,"* rather than the patient (the terrain). This antiquated theory groomed to maturity, bore the most elaborate and deadly premeditated hoax of all time, allowing the *"business with disease"* to endlessly perpetuate the disease industry. It solidifies the requirement for complexity so necessary for industry growth and preservation.

The hoax has been perpetuated for over a century and a half now. It is referred to as ***"traditional medicine."*** Most practicing physicians are completely oblivious to the fact that they are part of the hoax, for it is all they know, have ever been taught, and reinforcement by the establishment in the protection of their multi-trillion dollar investment with disease is formidable.

By *embracing* the germ theory and de-emphasizing the importance of the terrain, the patient's and society's focus in general is insulated from prevention through cellular nutrition, to **a reliance on *The System*** when health problems inevitably arise. The cause and effect philosophy serves to keep the answers to health complex, above the comprehension of the common man. The introduction of the Greek/Latin language in medicine served to further keep the patient standing on the outside looking in.

Conversely, the importance of *the terrain* or *bodily environment* (prevention through proper cellular nutrition and care) is an easy concept for the public to grasp, and happens to be the inconvenient truth (for the system) of optimum health.

In 1860, Florence Nightingale often referred to as *the founder of modern nursing,* enlightened many to the fact that *"Nature alone cures."* She understood the very basis of healing, even though technology was in a state of infancy in her day. She stated that, *"Pathology* (The study of disease, Ed.) *teaches the harm that disease has done. But it teaches nothing more. We know nothing of the principle of health, the positive of which pathology is the negative, except from observation and experience. And nothing but observation and experience will teach us the ways to maintain or to bring back the state of health. It is often thought that medicine is the curative process. It is no such thing; medicine is the surgery of functions, as surgery proper is that of limbs and organs. Neither can do anything but remove obstructions; neither can cure; nature alone cures. Surgery removes the bullet out of the limb, which is an obstruction to cure, but nature heals the wound. So it is with medicine; the function of an organ becomes obstructed; medicine, so far as we know, assists nature to remove the obstruction, but does nothing more. ... If I have succeeded in any measure in dispelling this illusion, and in showing what true nursing is, and what it is not, my object will have been answered."*

She further stated: *"The specific disease doctrine (the germ theory) is the grand refuge of weak, uncultured, unstable minds, such as now rule in the medical profession. There are no specific diseases; **there are specific disease conditions.**"* In recognition of her brilliant work, Queen Victoria awarded Nightingale the Royal Red Cross in 1883. Our hats are certainly off to her courage and brilliance today.

Dr. Virginia Vetrano: *"Hygienists object to the germ theory of disease because germs do not cause disease. They may be present in disease processes, and they many complicate a disease with their waste products which can be very toxic at times, but the germ or virus alone is never the sole cause of disease."*

Dr. Robert R. Goss; *"Germs do not cause disease! Nature never surrounded her children with enemies. It is the individual himself who* *makes disease possible in his own body because of poor living habits . . . Do mosquitoes make the water stagnant; or does stagnant water attract the mosquitoes? We should all be taught that <u>germs are friends and scavengers attracted by disease,</u> rather {than} enemies <u>causing disease</u> . . . <u>As their internal environment is, so will be the</u> attraction <u>for any specific micro-organism</u> . . . <u>The germ theory and</u> vaccination <u>are kept going by commercialism.</u>"*

Let it be clearly understood that *The Establishment's Multi- Trillion Dollar Hoax* **continues today, at the expense of your health.**

Always *"Searching for The Cures,"* …but where *are* the cures?

Much of the *"cure image"* enjoyed by Big Pharma today was originally created from the initial success of antibiotics and vaccines which were touted as *"wonder-drugs."* Two generations later we now have *"Superbugs"* resistant to antibiotics and a staggering increase in every major disease.

What actually caused the reduction or elimination of most of infectious diseases, such as polio, smallpox, rheumatic and scarlet fever, dysentery, etc.? Was it antibiotics, vaccines and *"wonder-drugs"* as we have been led to believe? According to Leonard Horowitz, PhD, a Harvard graduate in Public Health and Tufts University in Dentistry, <u>it was due to improved public sanitation, modern plumbing, and garbage disposal.</u> He documents declining rates of these diseases before the use of these vaccinations. He also implicates rising rates of autism, neurological disorders, and cancer after the introduction of mass vaccination. The State of California has the highest rate of autism as well as the highest vaccination rate.

The concept of vaccinations is to build up the immunity for a particular disease causing organism. By injecting weakened, dead, or attenuated bacteria or viral particles along with *adjuvants* (chemicals that may stimulate an immune response), an immunity may be built up. This immunity is often less powerful and of shorter duration than naturally acquired immunity and the adjuvants and other additives such as formaldehyde and mercury may be quite harmful. This danger increases with multiple vaccinations as these toxins accumulate. According to the National Vaccination Foundation, the state of California with the highest levels of vaccinations has the highest rate of autism which has been implicated with mercury poisoning.

It is the immune system that recognizes the invading organism where upon the next exposure, it can be dealt with effectively without the need for medications. The same is true of vaccinations which, when they work, do so because they stimulate immune response. Even when vaccines are effective they are often less so than a naturally acquired immunity from exposure to the offending organism. Curiously once again, when the patient is allowed to remain in low resistance from absence of health through cellular support, the market for vaccines is enormous.

Antibiotics have been abused and overused for decades now. Where upon once a simple dosage of penicillin would eliminate most common infections in a few days, now it is typical to prescribe much more powerful and potentially dangerous antibiotics for two weeks or longer in much higher doses. This over-prescribing of antibiotics has created a growing list of superbugs such as Methacillin Resistant Staphylococcus Aureus (MRSA), E. coli, and Pseudomonas species as well as many others.

There is a growing list of diseases, once relatively rare, now increasing at alarming rates. Rates are continuing to rise for mostly preventable diseases such as Type 2 diabetes, autism, heart disease, and cancer. I recall reading an article appearing in a local Long-Island newspaper in the late 70's which documented a statement by an international meeting of cancer researchers at Cold Spring Harbor Research Laboratories hosted by Dr's Watson and Crick (Nobel prize winners who had described the structure of DNA) concluding that, "If people improved their diets, there would likely be a 50% decrease in cancer and if we also "cleaned up the environment," we would probably eliminate 75% of all cancers." They went on to say that they were conservatively trained scientists, and therefore, they "purposely underestimated these figures." Approximately eighty percent of diabetics will die prematurely from cardiovascular disease. It has recently been estimated that one out of two, to one out of three American children alive today will develop diabetes within their lifetime. Diabetes is the leading cause of blindness, kidney disease, circulatory disease, and amputations. One out of two Americans will develop cardiovascular disease and one out of three will develop cancer.

One may argue that interferon treatment for Hepatitis C is a cure but this treatment has so many severe side effects that only approximately 50% of the patients make it through the year long treatment program. Even after this arduous and extremely expensive program, many patients are left with persistent viral counts and therefore face the uncertain future of the infection flaring up again. Like virtually every other infection, many persons exposed to the hepatitis C virus never develop the condition, due to a strong and healthy immune system.

The public is under the impression that the pharmaceutical industry has and is continuing to invent cures for disease. *We are hard-pressed to think of one.* Even antibiotics when used appropriately will not cure anyone of any infection, unless their immune system is functioning, because while antibiotics inhibit the replication of bacteria, ultimately it is the immune system which will destroy the last surviving bacteria. In addition, as discussed, antibiotics may also destroy friendly bacteria needed for digestion as well as promote super-infections when over-prescribed or not used properly.

As discussed, most, if not all pharmaceutical medications *treat symptoms,* not the cause of disease. For example, non-steroidal anti-inflammatory drugs such as aspirin, acetaminophen, ibuprophen, etc., are designed to reduce certain inflammatory pathways. Unfortunately, they also inhibit cartilage producing cells (chondrocytes) from producing cartilage. So you see, nothing is done to stop the *cause* of the inflammation, and the side effect further exacerbates the problem (arthritis with loss of cartilage). The more powerful antiinflammatory drugs such as cortisone, prednisone, methotrexate, etc., have even more severe side effects such as **immune suppression,** adrenal insufficiency, fluid retention, and hormonal disturbances. None of these cure any disease, they only treat symptoms, and at best give *temporary pain relief* until hopefully the body can cure or heal itself. This happens only if and when the body, and in particular the immune system, is in a strong enough state to do so! (cellular support).

Diuretics, taken to treat high blood pressure may temporarily lower blood pressure, but with prolonged use will often damage the kidney. Kidney damage leads to high blood pressure! So here again, the treatment eventually exacerbates the problem, often calling for more drugs or surgical intervention such as kidney dialysis, heart, kidney, or liver transplants. The long-term use of these high tech band-aids are dangerous, exorbitantly expensive, and deleterious to the quality and length of life.

An Attitude Revealed

Here is an astounding fact that sheds direct light on the *attitude* of the Modern Medicine System. Under Medicare, maintenance care called, *"Maintenance Therapy"* is excluded from coverage! "Maintenance Therapy" under Medicare is defined as: *"Services that seek to prevent disease, promote health, and prolong and enhance the quality of life; or maintain or prevent deterioration of a chronic condition."* These are **not** considered **"medically necessary"** under Medicare, and therefore, are not reimbursable! We would present the question: What on earth could possibly be more important to the overall health and welfare of the American people other than "maintenance therapy" as described above; namely, the prevention of disease, the promotion of health, the enhancement of the quality of life, and prevention of deterioration caused by chronic disease? It would seem that their philosophy is; *just wait for them to develop disease, and when they do, we'll attempt to patch them up at the twelfth hour.*

Obviously, maintenance therapy should be *encouraged,* not discouraged! The assurance of the essential phytonutrients and healing components, which enable cellular function and communication within our bodies to operate at an optimum level, is obviously the single most important aspect of maintenance therapy. We must allow our bodies to remain in a state conducive to natural healing, for as Florence Nightingale so eloquently stated; *"nature alone cures."*

Critical Health Information
Withheld or Inaccurate

We cannot count the number of times which we have had a patient announce that their medical doctor has told them that *"the supplementation of vitamins and minerals is a waste of money,"* and the most famous cliché; *"it will just turn your urine yellow and end up in the toilet."* Possibly the reader has heard this as well. Could there be a more clinically ignorant statement come out of the mouth of a "health care provider?" It is as if they received a notice from the AMA saying; *"Just tell the patient this."* We already know prevention is not on their menu, but how about a little common sense. How many research studies does it take before they wake up to the facts concerning what the body needs to function and that these nutrients just are not in our foods in any significant amount any longer? According to the AMA, the average individual absorbs less than 10% of synthetic vitamins. But instead of instructing the doctors to inform the patients of the need to supplement with organic nutrient sources, they seem to simply state a half-truth and leave the patient misinformed, cellularly malnourished, and thus susceptible to disease. Another damaging piece of *"advice"* remains one of their favorites; *"Eating a balanced diet will provide you with all the vitamins and minerals you need."* This is of course, virtually impossible given our nutrient deficient food supply, evidenced by the rising rates of disease.

Due to today's poor nutritional quality of food in general, we all certainly need to supplement with organic phytonutrients, vitamins, minerals, and immune modulators on a daily basis. The absorption potential of these "designed for the body" nutrients is extremely high in most individuals. Even if an individual initially has poor absorption capabilities, some percentage of the supplement will be absorbed and utilized by the body while the modulators restore absorption. Should something *"end up in the toilet,"* so be it! Everything we ingest ends up in the toilet after the body has taken what it needs or is able to absorb. Should we stop eating all together because some percentage of our nutrients ends up in the toilet? Of course not! This type of industry rhetoric is an obvious and pathetic attempt to shift the patient's focus from prevention to relying on drugs and after-the-fact (illness) "care." It is a stark indication that doctors may utter *almost anything* without question, if instructed from those above, due to their perception of establishment infallibility.

The fact that this auto-dissemination of misinformation by *"health care professionals"* is still going on today is amazing for numerous reasons, but how profound is it considering the fact that the AMA was almost forced to reverse their policy on vitamin and mineral intake in 2002?

The Journal of the American Medical Association published an article entitled *"Vitamins for Chronic Disease Prevention in Adults,"* June 19, 2002 Vol. 287, No. 23. Upon reading the article in its entirety, it becomes obvious that it is a self-serving attempt to further confuse. In opinion, the basic purpose of the article was to quasi-acknowledge the mountains of research supporting vitamin supplementation in a pretentious effort to put forth the impression that *"the subject has been reviewed,"* while continuing to confuse and therefore discourage doctors from recommending nutritional supplements and to continue the establishment's long standing opposition to natural prevention.

We have included an excerpt from the article below. In the midst of much double talk and common-sense avoidance, some astounding and long understood conclusions were admitted;

Drs. Robert H. Fletcher and Kathleen M. Fairfield of Harvard University, who wrote JAMA's *"new guidelines"* (They're guiding us) concluded;

"Inadequate intake of several vitamins has been linked to chronic diseases, *including* coronary heart disease, cancer, and osteoporosis."

Let's read that last sentence again!!

For decades the medical establishment has been telling us that vitamins are *"a waste of money."*

The last time JAMA made a comprehensive review of vitamins, about 25 years ago, it concluded people of normal health should not take multivitamins because they were *"a waste of time and money."*

While they have sent us off in the wrong direction over the last several decades, heart disease, cancer, osteoporosis, and birth defects, among many other diseases, have risen to alarming rates. These "rates" involve peoples' lives. Millions of people have presumably suffered and died because of the dissemination of this misinformation. Even today, after the publication of this *"reversal in policy,"* according to numerous patients, medical doctors are still telling their patients vitamins and minerals are *"a waste of money and end up in the toilet."* They are still telling us that they do not understand the *"cause"* of these *"incurable diseases,"* and yet the mountains of scientific research state that the evidence points to a lack of supporting phytonutrients.

Centers for Disease Control and Prevention: *"Current evidence collectively demonstrates that fruit and vegetable intake is associated with improved health, reduced risk of major diseases, and possibly delayed onset of age-related factors."*

We cannot turn on the television without being bombarded with pharmaceutical advertisements claiming to be the solution for everything. They tell us to *"ask our doctor"* about every concoction marketed as if they are the solutions for our ailments.

What is going on in *"health care?"* Why are medical doctors not informing, instructing, or urging the public to initiate and stay on specific nutritional supplementation regimens, in an effort to prevent an entire array of potential diseases? What is going on with the dissemination of valuable health information among our *"health care professionals"* and the modern medical system? Where is the trust?

Big Pharma pressures are behind the withholding of this critical information to the public. A healthy public is not conducive for large pharmaceutical sale volumes. They claim to be in search of *"the magic bullets"* when in reality they seem to be doing everything possible to hide them, because the real magic bullets are natural and cannot be patented. Instead, they aggressively market their toxic bullets which are clearly killing us. They are killing over 100,000 of us each year and damaging potentially millions more while attempting to convince us that vitamins and minerals are dangerous and that God does not really know what he is doing.

Linus Pauling, two-time Nobel Prize scientist stated that heart disease could be prevented using nutritional therapy especially vitamin C. We make an example of the following studies, conducted in 1939 to illustrate that the suppression of information has indeed been going on for decades. **Today, diabetes is striking one out of three Americans and heart disease is affecting 50%.**

As stated by Matthias Rath, M.D. in his 2001 book, *"The Heart";* Clinical studies show that vitamin C in diabetic patients not only contributes to prevention of cardiovascular complications, but also helps to normalize the imbalance in the glucose metabolism.

Professor R. Pfleger and his colleagues from the University of Vienna published the results of a remarkable clinical study. They showed that diabetic patients taking from 300 to 500 milligrams of vitamin C daily could significantly improve glucose balance. Blood sugar levels could be lowered on average by 30%, daily insulin requirements by 27%, and sugar excretion in the urine could be almost eliminated. It is amazing that this study was published in 1937 in a leading European journal for internal medicine. If the results of this important study had been followed up with further research and documented in medical textbooks, millions of lives may have been saved and cardiovascular disease would have been greatly reduced among diabetic patients and the rest of us as well.

Another study conducted at Stanford University in California conducted by Dr. J.F. Dice, went on to show that for every additional gram of dietary vitamin C supplementation, Dr. Dice could reduce the patients dosage by about 2 units of insulin.

Despite the fact that there is a huge and ever increasing volume of documented scientific evidence supporting the critical nature of adequate nutrient intake in regard to preventing, fighting, and eliminating disease, published by some of the most prestigious medical journals in the world, including The New England Journal of Medicine, The Journal of the American Medical Association, and The American Journal of Clinical Nutrition, the medical establishment persists in their long-standing policy to largely ignore these findings. How do we get the doctors to read their own journals? It is almost impossible to find a doctor who will share this critical information with the patient. Few are willing to step outside the box. With seemingly little choice, they continue to perpetuate the drug industries view of nutrition as the enemy rather than the ally in the prevention and elimination of disease.

Interestingly, in most cases when the patient brings up the subject of good health and prevention through proper nutrition, medical doctors will agree and not dispute the findings of the patient. Yet in the overwhelming majority of cases, they will not do what we would expect of the health care professional. Most will not be initially forthcoming with the vital information regarding nutrition unless first confronted by an educated patient. Even if he *"agrees,"* the physician's effort to pursue a nutritional program for the patient seems to begin and end with a few comments such as; *"Oh that's fine."* or ... *"That can't hurt you,"* etc. These empty comments are designed to be non-confrontational as to not risk the loss of the patient.

Can you remember the last time your doctor looked you square in the eye and told you; *"Listen carefully to me now. Adequate intake of vital nutrients has been shown to prevent and eliminate an entire host of degenerative diseases, so we need to get you on a good supervised program to ensure your quality of life and longevity?"*

This anti-natural-solution *policy* stands in an effort to perpetuate drug-profits and medical procedures made *"necessary"* by largely *preventable* widespread illness. Once again, the system is self-preserving.

If we are *informed,* healthy, and free from ailments and disorders, we would not need to "ask our doctor about" ...Any drugs!

What's the Mystery?

There are cultures of peoples existing in the world today where disease is almost non-existent. They suffer almost no degenerative disease at all, while living a vigorous lifestyle to ages often exceeding 100 years. Although difficult to document with any degree of precision, some claim many individuals within these cultures live to the 130 – 140 range. They are the Armenians between Iran and Turkey, the Hunzas of Eastern Pakistan, the Okinawians, the Tibetans of Western China, the Titicacas on the Peru-Bolivian border, and the Vilcabamba Indians in the Andes Mountains of Ecuador.

These cultures do not have doctors or drugs, yet on average, they live decades longer than Americans, and their aging (degeneration) process is dramatically slower. All of these cultures have a few other obvious things in common as well. Their food sources are rich with phytonutrients, grown in nutrient-rich, uncontaminated soils. Their water supplies contain extremely high levels of minerals, and they consume many times our *"Recommended Daily Allowances"* (RDA) of all vitamins and minerals. These facts are widely known among the scientific community, which is generally decades ahead of the traditional medical community, apparently both by choice.

There are those who suspect, the authors inclusive, that our RDA's are set purposely low with the full understanding by some that the consumption of these low levels of nutrients will indeed leave us vulnerable to the entire gamut of diseases. Remember, pharmaceuticals are not used or needed in the healthiest cultures in the world. If we were informed enough to mimic their habits of consumption, pharmaceuticals, one of the largest and most powerful industries on earth, would dwindle to obscurity.

The current recommended daily allowances (RDA's) of vitamins and minerals are set by the governing bodies at such a ridiculously low benchmark, that they encourage the development and proliferation of disease through deficiency. Science shows us that those who ingest low levels are the sickest among Americans.

Doctors are trained by establishment authorities who are influenced by Big Pharma to disseminate this type of misinformation to their patients, which subsequently perpetuates their ill-health. Can you imagine the drug industry encouraging doctors to prescribe natural preventions and cures rather than their economically lucrative drugs? In most cases, medical doctors have only a few hours of training in nutritional therapy. This shocking atrocity is due in large to the drug industry's influence on medical curriculum. True *healthcare* through targeted nutrition is the *opposite* direction in which modern medicine is forcibly focused. It is the enemy of the *business with disease.*

The Invasion of The Health Snatchers

As a society, we have become the host for parasitic pharmaceutical and medical procedural profits. Americans consume 50% of the prescription pharmaceuticals and 60% of the psychiatric drugs in the world. At 5% of the world population this means Americans take 10X's the drugs and 12X's the psychiatric drugs as compared to the rest of the world. Those softly-lit, beautifully flowing drug-ads seem to be hitting their mark. Given these numbers, quite obviously, their marketing efforts have been successful. Americans have been *"asking their doctors"* about everything except *the real answers to health.* But in truth, why should the public be *forced* to *ask* when a *medical professional* is paid, and more importantly, possesses the **trust** of the patient to provide these answers automatically?

What's in *Your* Wallet?

According to The National Coalition on Health Care (NCHC), the United States spends more per person on health care than any other country, yet in overall quality its care ranks a shameful 37th in the world, according to a World Health Organization analysis. In 2005, health care spending in the United States reached *2 trillion dollars,* and was projected to reach 2.9 trillion in 2009. Health care spending was then projected to reach 4 trillion by 2015. We as a society have become the unsuspecting host. Health care spending is 4.3 times the amount spent on national defense. Only through education, awareness, and good common sense can we defend ourselves against this insidious parasite preying upon the people of our homeland; the current Pharma/Medical *"healthcare"* establishment.

The promotion of preventative medicine, through a focus on optimum cellular health will lead to the cure for America's current plague of degenerative diseases, save us billions, possibly our economy and country, and both lengthen and dramatically improve the quality of our lives.

The mission of this book, *"The Code of Life..."* is to provide One Giant Step in that magnificent direction.

Chapter 6

The Amazing
Immune System

In our environment, we are continuously exposed to substances that are *capable* of causing us harm. The skin acts as one physical barrier to many potentially invading organisms. We also have a more advanced protective system called *the immune system.*

The immune system is a complex network of organs containing cells designed to recognize foreign substances within the body and destroy them. The immune system protects us against pathogens or infectious agents such as viruses, bacteria, fungi, and parasites. The human immune system is the most complex and widely distributed system throughout the entire human body.

The immune system is responsible for protecting us from disease. It is of such fundamental importance to our health that it will continue to function even after most other systems have failed and it will even break down other tissues to maintain its functions. Therefore anemia (diminished hemoglobin or red cells in the blood) can cause one to feel "run down" and to have a "lowered resistance." During an infection, the body can break down the red blood cells' hemoglobin into heme (iron) and globin (globulin), the protein component with immune function, which your body can then reassemble to form immunoglobulins (as in gamma globulin). The red cells act as a store of this globulin, which can be recycled into other immune components. Thus illustrated, the immune system is of such critical importance, it is designed to take priority in times of crisis (i.e. specific nutrient deficiency) over other systems of the body.

There are two major divisions of the immune system. The first produces antibodies from the liver and lymphocytes. These antibodies are liquid proteins that circulate in the bloodstream and throughout other body fluids. These substances interfere with the growth of pathogens (infectious agents which cause disease or illness) or clump them together so that they can be recognized and later destroyed by immune cells called phagocytes. This is the *humoral immunity system.* The second is referred to as the *cellular immunity system* which produces cells such as macrophages and killer T-cells which migrate throughout the body on patrol for harmful invaders. There are various immune cells such as polymorphonuclear leukocytes (white cells), macrophages (cells which ingest and digest foreign substances, bacteria, and toxins), eosinophiles, and mast cells that fight parasites and allergies, and natural killer cells that destroy viruses and certain cancer cells. This cellular immune system produces cells that engulf and destroy bacteria, viruses, fungi, parasites, cancer cells, and cellular debris from injuries and infections. Without these mobile defenders we would be vulnerable to virtually anything entering the body and the simplest virus or bacteria would be able to multiply rapidly and become fatal.

Substances capable of generating an immune response are called antigens. Antigens are not the foreign microorganisms and tissues themselves; they are substances found on or within them that can be recognized by the immune system and for which antibodies can be produced. Immune responses are normally directed against the antigen that provoked them and are said to be antigen-specific. Because of this recorded response, once you are exposed to a harmful microorganism or toxin, you will henceforth possess a cellular memory which will fight that particular offender in the future. This is also known as "immunologic memory." Immunologic memory is the ability of the immune system to mount a stronger and more effective immune response against an antigen after its first encounter with that antigen, leaving us better able to resist future attacks. In perspective; infants born with immune system failure do not survive. Our health in general is directly correlated to the overall strength and efficiency of our immune systems.

Lymphocytes are made from stem cells in the bone marrow which undergo several stages of development in the acquisition of their antigen-specific receptors. In developing fetuses, lymphocytes are made in the liver. Lymphocytes which are processed in the bone marrow are called B-cells. These immune surveillance cells migrate to other areas of the body. B-cells are lymphocytes that play a large role in the humoral immune response as opposed to the cell-mediated immune response that is governed by T-cells. The principle function of B-cells is to make antibodies against antigens. B-cells are an essential component of the adaptive immune system.

It is the adaptive immune response that provides our immune system with the ability to recognize and remember specific pathogens and to mount stronger attacks each time the pathogen is encountered. This is termed *"adaptive"* immunity because the body's immune system is preparing itself for future challenges.

Other lymphocytes move from the bone marrow and are processed in the thymus, a pyramid-shaped lymphoid organ located immediately beneath the breastbone at the level of the heart. These lymphocytes are called T-lymphocytes, or T-cells (thymus-derived cells).

An antibody is used by the immune system to identify and neutralize foreign objects like bacteria and viruses. Antibodies attack antigens by binding to them. Some antibodies attach themselves to invading microorganisms and render them immobile or prevent them from penetrating healthy cells. In other cases, the antibodies act together with a group of blood proteins collectively called the complement system that consists of at least 30 different components. In such cases, antibodies coat the antigen and make it subject to a chemical chain reaction with the complement proteins. The complement reaction either can cause the invader to burst or can attract scavenger cells that "eat" the invader.

There are two major classes of T-cells produced in the thymus: helper T-cells and killer T-cells. Helper T-cells secrete molecules called interleukins (IL) that promote the growth of both B and T-cells. Normally these immune stimulating interleukins are made in response to invading organisms. In those with weakened immune systems, this process may be defective. Fortunately, Interleukin II is stimulated by the long chain polymannans found in Aloe. For a person experiencing weakened immunity, which may be all of us to varying degrees, the ingestion of these polymannans can be lifesaving. The interleukins are secreted by lymphocytes which are also called lymphokines. The interleukins that are secreted by other kinds of blood cells called monocytes and macrophages are called monokines. Some ten different interleukins are known: IL-1, IL-2, IL-3, IL-4, IL-5, IL-6, IL-7, interferon, lymphotoxin, and tumor necrosis factor. Each interleukin has complex biological effects.

Cytotoxic t-cells belong to a sub-group of T-lymphocytes (a type of white blood cell) which are capable of inducing the death of infected somatic (body) or tumor cells; they kill cells that are infected with viruses (or other pathogens), or are otherwise damaged or dysfunctional. Cytotoxic T-cells are also called suppressor lymphocytes because they regulate immune responses by suppressing the function of helper cells so that the immune system is active only when necessary. Aloe glucomannans stimulate the production of killer T-cells. It has been shown that the glucomannans from Aloe stimulate the production of lymphoid (immune) tissues and thereby increase immune function. They stimulate the production of Interleukin II boosting immune function. Glucomannans also increase the production of killer T-cells, so vitally important in fighting bacteria and viruses.

The most powerful immune enhancing Aloe-derived components are the long and very long chain polymannans (Acemannan), which, to be preserved, must be prepared carefully as they will break down by the action of enzymes, heat or acid. Dr. Borecky and Associates in 1967 authored a paper entitled, *"An Interpheron-Like Substance Induced by Mannans."* Interpheron is an antiviral substance. Synthetic Interpheron is currently being used to treat hepatitis "C", but the synthetic has so many side effects that only approximately 50% of those prescribed it finish the year long treatment. There is no known toxicity or any dangerous side-effects from the ingestion of the Aloe polymannans. In 1990, Dr. Kemp demonstrated antiviral properties against HIV, Newcastle disease, and influenza with the use of polymannans. Improved survival rates of cats with feline leukemia were shown by Dr. Yates and Associates in 1992 with the use of the polymannans. The work of Pulse & Uhlig in 1990 showed that all 29 HIV-positive patients in the study improved by 90 days. Their quality of life scores increased from 78.9% to 92.41%. Decreased infectivity was demonstrated against the AIDS virus, Newcastle disease, and herpes simplex virus in a study by Dr. Kahion in 1991.

Targeted cellular and immune support can restore health in a rapid fashion. A man entered my office in a wheelchair, complaining of difficulty walking with lower back pain. After I had eliminated his back pain and he no longer needed the wheelchair, I questioned him further regarding his general health. He revealed to me that he was HIV positive for fourteen years and was suffering from severe weight loss, chronic diarrhea, and fatigue. He had red blotches over most of his body and was severely depressed. I asked him if he would like to try something natural that would help him with these problems. He was quite receptive and began taking the immune modulating components. Three days later, his chronic diarrhea disappeared. Three weeks later, the red blotches were gone, his killer T-cell count had risen over thirty percent and he gained five pounds which he desperately needed. He had a marked increase in energy and his spirits were noticeably elevated. The last time I saw him a year later, he was continuing to feel well.

The receptors of T-cells are different from those of B-cells because they are "trained" to recognize fragments of antigens that have been combined with a set of molecules found on the surfaces of all the body's cells. As T-cells circulate throughout the body, they scan the surfaces of body cells for the presence of foreign antigens. This function is sometimes referred to as *immune surveillance.*

Immune surveillance is the term used to describe the cells of the immune system which are in constant circulation about the body. Whenever these cells come in contact with anything recognized as foreign, they will attempt to destroy it. As discussed, there are polysaccharides (including components from polymannans) that attach to the surfaces of these cells. These polysaccharide identifiers are used by other cells to recognize self from foreign. It is essential that this recognition process be as accurate as possible so that our own cells are not misread by these circulating immune cells and thereby attacked as in autoimmune disease (self-attacking-self). The restoration of the accurate recognition process which guides the immune system to see and eliminate the harmful foreign invaders, also prevents the immune system form attacking self (the cells, tissues and organs of the body).

Now you understand how the root-cause, driving-force of over 100 autoimmune diseases, all classified as "incurable" by the Drug Cartel, is progressively eliminated by natural immune modulating components.

Immune surveillance is also believed to be one of the primary ways your immune system recognizes a cancer cell. It is also believed that even in healthy individuals, cancer cells are being created, but immune surveillance works to destroy these abnormal cells before they mutate enough to become a problem.

The lack of sufficient phytonutrient and specific complex carbohydrate substances in the modern diet is contributing to the breaking down or weakening of our immune systems. Our experiences, and strong scientific evidence demonstrates that we are able to avoid, or at the very least minimize, the devastating consequences of autoimmune and degenerative diseases by supplementing our diet with these natural healing nutrients.

Chapter 7

The Functions of the Carbohydrates making up the *"Symbols"* of The Code

Research into carbohydrates has revealed they are far reaching and very important structural and metabolic functions. These include among many others, glycogen for energy storage, ribose, and deoxy-ribose in nucleic acids (DNA and RNA which make up the genetic code), metabolic intermediates (for energy production), glycolipids in cell membranes and the nervous system, glycoproteins in the immune system, proteoglycans in cartilage and collagen found in connective tissues throughout the body. Science has also firmly established the importance of these carbohydrate molecules in their relationship to cellular communication; reinforcing what has been observed for thousands of years, *Aloe enhanced healing.* These carbohydrates are either essential components of, directly or indirectly control, regulate, or influence the vital processes of digestion, reproduction, healing, immunity, cellular, and tissue repair. These carbohydrates are critical to virtually every cell, tissue, and organ within our body.

Some examples of the many forms of these complex carbohydrates and their functions are: glycosaminoglycans (mucopolysaccharides) which protect the respiratory, gastrointestinal, and urinary tracts. These coat the mucous membranes that are so important for protecting us from bacteria, viruses, fungi, parasites, and other foreign invaders such as dust and pollen. They also form proteoglycans which are incorporated into cartilage which cushions, lubricates, and protects our joints. The popular nutritional supplements chondroitin sulfate and glucosamine sulfate used by many today for the prevention or alleviation of arthritis are made from these carbohydrate molecules. These carbohydrates attach themselves to the protein surface of each cell and function as the symbols which communicate a language from cell to cell. Without these symbols there is no communication between cells. Without these symbols we are defenseless against chronic disease.

The Glycocalyx, or *"The Fuzz"*

The list is virtually endless in relation to where these essential carbohydrates are found. Hyaluronic acid is found in sperm and the intervertebral discs of the spine. Heparin which is essential for proper blood clotting, glycoproteins, and glycolipids occur in cell membranes and serum albumin (the major protein found in the liquid portion of the blood) also contains these essential carbohydrates. Glycolipids and gangliosides are essential components of the nervous system. The presence of these glycoproteins on the outer surface of the plasma membrane (the glycocalyx or *the fuzz*) covers cell surfaces for important cellular recognition, communication, and other immunological functions. In healthy cells, so omnipresent are these carbohydrate molecules that cells appear to other cells and to the immune system as covered in a blanket of fuzz. Cells communicate through their own language of chemical signals. Once the signal chemical binds to a receptor, that protein turns on a signaling cascade in the cell that ultimately leads to the cell's response. This cell-surface "fuzz" contains an integral part of The Code of Life for cellular communication.

Galactose is needed for the synthesis of lactose (milk sugar), glycolipids, proteoglycans, and glycoproteins. Galactose is readily converted in the liver to glucose. Your body can make glucose from galactose. Galactose is required in the body as a constituent of proteoglycans, glycoproteins, and glycolipids (the cerebrosides of the nervous system). Cerebrosides are components that make up the insulation surrounding the nerves known as the *myelin sheath.* Multiple sclerosis (MS) is an example of a disease in which the glycolipid, the insulating material coating the nerves, is defective. Multiple sclerosis affects neurons, the cells of the brain and spinal cord that carry information, create thought and perception, and allow the brain to control the entire body. Surrounding and protecting some of these neurons is this fatty myelin sheath layer, which helps neurons carry electrical signals. Multiple sclerosis causes gradual destruction of the myelin sheath (demyelination) and transection (cuts into the coating of the nerves) of neuron axons in patches throughout the brain and spinal cord. The name *multiple sclerosis* refers to the multiple scars (or scleroses) on the myelin sheaths. This scarring causes neurological symptoms which vary widely depending upon which signals are interrupted.

One of the major amino sugars is glucosamine, a major component of cartilage. This is an example of a glycoprotein. The body produces glucosamine, an essential component of healthy cartilage from glucose and amino acids. These complex carbohydrates are incorporated into cell membranes. Glycophingolipids are sugar containing lipids. They are located in the plasma membranes of cells. Many of the proteins and all of the glycolipids have externally exposed oligosaccharide chains.

The Biochemistry of
Cellular Communication

Complex carbohydrate chains, when available, attach to cell surfaces and are the means through which one cell communicates with another. This type of cell to cell communication is referred to as intercellular communication. Although much is yet to be discovered in regard to this miraculous phenomenon, we presently know that variations in the configurations of these complex carbohydrates determine how our own cells recognize each other, and how they recognize a foreign cell. This cellular recognition is an essential immune function because the cells of the immune system must recognize and destroy disease causing organisms while leaving our own cells intact and undamaged. Autoimmune diseases are partially due to a breakdown of this function. *Autoimmunity* is the failure of an organism to recognize its own constituent parts (down to the cellular level) as *"self"*, which results in an immune response (an attack) against its own cells and tissues. Without adequate amounts of these essential carbohydrates the immune system cannot function properly. One of the many remarkable actions of these immunologically active substances from Aloe is their "immune modulatory" effects. Immune modulation refers to a regulatory or balancing function, not just a stimulatory one.

All the physiological actions which are constantly maintaining normal function must remain in balance. Just as we want a healthy and responsive immune system capable of recognizing and destroying abnormal cells, harmful bacteria, viruses, fungi, parasites, and toxins, we do not want an overactive immune system creating allergic, inflammatory, and self-destructive actions known as autoimmune disease. We do not want our hearts to beat too fast or too slow, too hard or too weakly. We want the food we eat to travel through our digestive tract at the required speed for optimal absorption of its nutritive value. We do not want our blood sugar to rise too far or too fast (diabetes) or fall too far or too fast (hypoglycemia). This regulatory process is known as homeostasis or *"balance."* These are just a few examples illustrating the critical importance of effective cell to cell communication.

I began working with a fourteen-year-old girl who was suffering with Type 1 Diabetes (insulin dependent). Her parents asked if there was anything that could be done to help stabilize her blood sugars for her insulin dosages were constantly being increased and were often too high or too low. Within three months on the stabilized immune modulators, we were able to stabilize her blood sugar levels (less highs and lows) and she was able to reduce her insulin to half of the previous dosage.

A fifty-year-old minister who was averaging blood sugars in the 200's (70-100 is considered normal), lowered his blood sugar readings to below 120 in three weeks using the immune modulators. He was so thrilled with the results he referred several of his parishioners to the program.

I was treating a husband and wife for chronic back pain who were both Type 2 diabetics. He was averaging a blood sugar level of over 200 and she was averaging over 300. Within six weeks on the modulators, both husband and wife had reduced their blood sugar counts by over 100 points each.

A nine-year-old boy who had been diagnosed with ulcerative colitis was brought into my office.

He was having up to a dozen bloody bowel movements per day. His pediatrician had placed him on medications including prednisone, 6- MP, Asacol, Flagyl, and other immunosuppressant drugs. The side effects of these drugs, some of which HE WAS EXPERIENCING, included swollen ankles, fatigue, and hair growing out of his forehead, a condition known as *hirsuitism*. He was missing school and unable to function normally while at school or at home. After three months of treatment with the modulators he was off all but one medication at a reduced dosage. His bowel movements became normal and were reduced to three daily with virtually no bleeding. He had no other symptoms whatsoever. He was playing normally, had returned to school, and was doing well.

In parallel to the existing scientific research on the immune modulators, we have had hundreds of other personal examples with patients recovering from autoimmune conditions (see many on DrRonPDrucker.com) and many thousands of recovery cases which we have been involved with by phone. The amazing part of the healing process with the modulators is that a physician can assist in healing a patient remotely by phone, and a patient can heal at home, in most cases, without any assistance from a physician.

Special Receptors Lying in Wait

Most common foods are broken down and absorbed by the typical processes of digestion. Conversely, there are specific essential complex carbohydrates or macromolecules which are required to be absorbed intact without being broken down or digested. These complex carbohydrates, known as Aloe polysaccharides or polymannans, are molecules linked together like beads in a necklace or links in a chain. The lengths of the chains vary and are responsible for the many diverse healing functions, including but not limited to, blood-sugar regulation, antioxidant functions, anti-inflammatory effects, wound healing, and immune modulation.

The human body is designed with special receptor sites called *enterons* which line the digestive tract. Miraculously, these special receptor sites are designed to take in or engulf, *intact,* these Aloe polymannans. This process is called *pinocytosis* or *endocytosis.*

Editor's note: As used here the term pinocytosis is interchangeable with the term endocytosis. Both terms refer to the process whereby large, undigested nutrient particles are taken into the enterons intact and unbroken, therefore being abundantly available for their many healing and nutritive purposes.

Due to this process these polymannans are absorbed in a totally different way which protects the links of the chains. The chains are not broken or digested by the digestive enzymes found in our digestive tract. These large chain macromolecules must be absorbed intact for their structure to retain their healing physiological functions. They must not be broken down by the digestive enzymes within the digestive tract so as to retain their healing properties. Therefore, this complimentary mechanism of endocytosis exists within the body to perform this essential task of absorption without destruction of these long chain structures.

The very existence of this complimentary process, these *"receptors in waiting,"* is indicative of the critical importance of the ingestion of these essential long chain macromolecules. **The human body, with these special receptor sites is literally lying in wait for these polymannan molecules.**

It is logical to assume that the human physiology was designed possessing these enterons to perform endocytosis or pinocytosis specifically to process these indigestible yet highly essential plant nutrients which had for millions of years been present in our food supply. Once inside the enteron, these macromolecules are carried to the sidewall of the cell where they are then introduced into the lymphatic system. From there they are transported to the bloodstream where they are carried to each and every cell in the body as required. At this stage, this miraculous process is referred to as *chemotaxis.* It is the transport of necessary cellular substances to the areas in need. In addition, in the presence of these macromolecules the process of chemotaxis is markedly enhanced!

Intracellular Communication

Once inside the cell, these long chain macromolecules which have been taken in by endocytosis including polysaccharides, polymannans proteins, and polynucleotides (DNA and RNA) can be used for their unique healing properties or broken down inside the cell for their nutritional value. We refer to this process as, *"intracellular digestion."* It is the second form of digestion which occurs *within* the cells. This form of digestion only occurs *after* these intact healing components have entered the interior of the cell where they are either utilized intact for their unique and necessary healing properties, or they may be broken down and processed into their subcomponents for further use.

The cell is composed of a cell membrane which surrounds the cytoplasm (the fluid inside the cell.) There are numerous organelles (cell organs) within the cell. An organelle is a discrete structure of a cell having specialized functions such as the mitochondria for energy production, the ribosomes for protein production, and the nucleus for cell replication.

There is a great deal of activity occurring within the cell. Communications of many types are taking place. For example, hormones have membrane receptors and use intracellular messengers to produce intracellular signals. The cells are virtual mini factories processing the spectrum of nutrients and producing energy, new cells, tissues (cell replication), and virtually every substance required for every physiologic function throughout the body.

The cells' semi-permeable outer membrane has channels that open to take in nutrients from the extracellular fluid such as the intestinal tract, lymph, or blood. These channels are opened by chemical messengers such as calcium ions, and hormones such as insulin which increases the transport of all nutrients into the cell interior. The cell can also excrete toxins, by-products of metabolism or manufactured substances that are needed elsewhere by the processes of channel transport for small molecules and by exocytosis for large macromolecules.

As mentioned, the cell is covered with a fuzzy coat called the glycocalyx made up of these essential carbohydrate and glycoprotein identifiers that direct the immune system to recognize self from foreign. Through this process of communication, immune cells may identify and destroy invaders or cells that have become defective, such as cancer cells, while leaving healthy cells unaffected.

Groups of cells organized together make up tissues, tissues form to make up organs, and the organs working in harmony permit the human body to perform its many various functions. The very basis of life, health, and longevity is healthy cells.

This complimentary digestive process of intracellular digestion is the process which fuels the cells. All essential nutrients must be available at all times for optimum cellular health and reproduction.

Optimum health depends on optimum cellular communication. "The Code of Life" is the language used for both intracellular (within the cell) and intercellular (cell to cell) communication. This cellular communication in whole enables virtually every physiological process within the body!

The Process of Exocytosis

Exocytosis is the process by which the cell releases macromolecules or expels toxins from the cell interior. Most cells release macromolecules such as proteins, antigens, and collagen to the exterior by exocytosis. The signal for exocytosis is often a hormone, which when it binds to a cell surface receptor induces a local transient change in calcium concentration. Hence, calcium *triggers* exocytosis. Hormones such as the glycoproteins, insulin and parathyroid hormone are also released by this calcium-reliant process. Calcium is also responsible for delivering nutrients into the cell, regulating cell membrane voltage and controlling channel openings which deliver vital nutrients into the cell's interior. Macromolecules, existing and entering the cell, which are too large to traverse these channel openings are transported within vesicles directly through the cell membrane.

The process of exocytosis involves the removal of toxins from the cells, transport of *intracellular* products, and *intercellular* communication, all of which are dependent upon healthy cell membranes. This exemplifies why the Aloe derived components are known to enhance detoxification.

Exocytosis is important in cellular signaling as well. In neuronal communication, both chemical and electrical information needs to be transmitted throughout the cell. Exocytosis sends and converts the electrical information into chemical information. Within the neural cells, the information is electrical. In the synapse (the gap between nerve cells) after exocytosis has occurred, the neurotransmitters are released and the information is chemical. The release of the neurotransmitter can either be excitatory (causing activity from the target cell) or inhibitory (preventing activity by the target cell).

Exocytosis is also needed by cells for secretion of proteins such as enzymes, peptide hormones, antibodies from cells, turnover of plasma membrane, release of neurotransmitter from presynaptic neurons, placement of integral membrane proteins, acrosome reaction (the release of hyaluronic acid to facilitate fertilization of the ovum by the spermatozoa) during fertilization, antigen presentation during the immune response, and recycling of plasma membrane bound receptors.

Other Important Functions
of the Essential Carbohydrates

Now that we have briefly explained the scientific details, one can readily understand why the ingestion of the complex carbohydrate components are so important to the vital functions related to them. The following is a partial list of the essential functions that are dependent upon or enhanced by their presence:

1) Reproduction
2) Nutrition
3) Immune function
4) Maintenance of normal blood sugar levels
5) Wound healing, cell and tissue regeneration
6) Detoxification including (exocytosis)
7) Anti-inflammatory functions
8) Antioxidant functions
9) Anti-aging functions

The partial list mentioned above encompasses several of the most important functions occurring within the body. Number five alone; *wound healing, cell and tissue regeneration* is the basis for healing. Remember, *We Are Cells – trillions of cells.* Health and healing begin at the cellular level.

Dr. Ivan Danhoff, recognized as one of the world's foremost experts on medically active plant molecules, states:

"The fact is that lining the gastrointestinal tract there are cells which are called enterons. These enterons are the lining cells of the digestive tract. Each of these cells produces a very sticky substance on the surface of their cells. This sticky substance is called the glycocalyx or sometimes it's just referred to as "the fuzz." It is in this glycocalyx that there are special receptors; special binding sites for the aloe polysaccharides. These binding sites or receptors are of two different types. The first type is called non-specific receptors and they bind the majority of the aloe polysaccharide which is taken into the body. When these polysaccharides are linked to these receptors it provides a marvelous protective action along the gastrointestinal tract. As a result of this protective function is one of the major things that can prevent the reflux of acid from your stomach into your esophagus. In fact, studies are currently being done now which show that the polysaccharides of aloe, with this binding to these non- specific receptors, may protect the lining of the esophagus from acid which is refluxed from the stomach. Now, in addition to these non- specific binding sites, there are specific binding sites or receptors. When these specific sites are bound to aloe polysaccharides a remarkable process occurs. The cell wall completely engulfs the polysaccharide, a process called pinocytosis or endocytosis. We find then that these aloe polysaccharides are now inside the cell (the enterocyte), the lining cell of the intestinal tract and they are then carried to the sidewall of the cell where they are then put into the lymphatic system and from the lymphatic system they are transported to the blood. So it means then by the special pinocytotic mechanism, the special cell engulfing mechanism, the aloe polysaccharides are able, even with very long chain lengths, to be transported across the lining of the intestinal tract and find their way into the bloodstream. We know then that this is a characteristic of polymannans and so the polymannans are handled by the digestive tract in this very special way; this process called pinocytosis."

Once again, Dr. Danhoff states: *"Now the aloe polysaccharide as we have indicated before may be of different lengths, so we have small necklaces, medium necklaces, large necklaces, and very long necklaces. As these lengths of chains of polysaccharides vary, we then find that there are a significant number of different healing activities."*

These essential carbohydrates also account for eight to ten percent of the weight of thyroglobulin (thyroid protein). The thyroid gland is one of the larger endocrine glands in the body. It is a double-lobed structure located in the neck, responsible for production of hormones that regulate the rate of metabolism and affect the growth and rate of function of many other systems in the body.

Erythropoietin is a glycoprotein which stimulates the production of red blood cells from the bone marrow. Red blood cells are the most common type of blood cell and the vertebrate (animals with backbones) body's principal means of delivering oxygen from the lungs to body tissues via the blood. Without adequate oxygen to the tissues, degeneration occurs and pain may be produced. A large number of other hematopoietic (production of blood cells) growth factors have been identified, most of which are glycoproteins. Like erythropoietin, most of the growth factors isolated have been glycoproteins, proving to be very active in-vivo (in live animals) and *in-vitro* (outside of a living organism such as in test tube or tissue culture), interacting with their target cells via specific cell surface receptors and ultimately (via intracellular signals) affecting vital *gene* expression.

The ABO substances (blood types) are complex oligosaccharides present in most cells of the body. The different saccharide molecules located at the end of these proteins determine blood types in humans. This is yet another example of how these carbohydrate molecules define and determine cellular recognition throughout all the tissues of the body.

Another interesting example is when a baby is born it is coated with a slick white layer of *Vernix*, also known as Vernix caseosa, which is the "waxy" or "cheesy" white substance, a mucopolysaccharide-rich protective coating. This facilitates delivery and is present to protect the infant from infection. These essential carbohydrates are necessary for the proper development of the fetus including the production of glycophingolipids, vital components of the nervous system.

The Difference Between
Simple and Complex Sugars

Simple sugars such as glucose (blood sugar), fructose (fruit sugar), sucrose (table, cane, or beet sugar), lactose (from dairy products), and maltose (from malt) are made up of short chains of carbon atoms to which are attached hydrogen and oxygen atoms. These are utilized for energy production and their caloric content. These sugars are in their simplest form and can be considered to be fuel or building blocks for the production of more complex forms. They are known as caloric sugars (sugars used for energy). These sugars should not be consumed in large amounts due to the fact that they require vitamins and minerals for their conversion to energy. Secondly, they stimulate the production of elevated insulin levels, obesity, the increased production of VLDL (very low density lipid), LDL (low density lipid, known as the "bad cholesterol"), and triglycerides. This is why we do not want to ingest large amounts of these particular types of *simple sugars.*

Conversely, *galactose* (synthesized by the body, forming glycolipids and glycoproteins in several tissues) and mannose are other variations of simple sugars which are not as readily available, and are not involved in the production of excess blood fats or triglycerides. Instead, they have been shown to possess an array of healing benefits. Complex carbohydrates are made up from these healing simple sugars. Two examples would be glycogen (stored in the liver and muscles) and starch, made up of long chains of glucose molecules attached to each other.

Complex carbohydrates include many types of fiber including indigestible cellulose, essential for normal bowel function and soluble fiber which has been found to lower cholesterol levels. Studies have found that consumption of adequate fiber lowers the incidence of bowel diseases including colon cancer.

Essential complex carbohydrates are involved with the maintenance of digestive function and normal blood-sugar levels, absorption of nutrients, destruction of disease causing organisms, the support and maintenance of friendly bacteria, regulation of inflammatory processes, and antioxidant functions.

Now we present the question, why, if new cells which make up every tissue and organ of the body are constantly being re-created does arthritis, autoimmune diseases, cancers, cardiovascular diseases, diabetes, ulcers, and other degenerative diseases remain and perpetuate? In the case of degenerative disease, what is it that is perpetuating the production of abnormal cells? Why are the cells continually reproducing in an abnormal fashion? What are they lacking that prevents them from reproducing in a normal and healthy state?

Science has repeatedly demonstrated that individuals suffering from chronic diseases are lacking in one or more essential nutrients, resulting in the cells' inability to function, reproduce, or communicate properly. With enhanced cellular communication and reproduction, many dysfunctions improve. This has been shown by significant improvement in blood sugar levels in diabetics and cholesterol and triglyceride levels in persons with elevated blood lipids.

Additional benefits include; the reduction of inflammation in arthritis, Crohn's disease and ulcerative colitis, improved wound healing, and the increase in immune cells and functions to mention just a few. Below we have listed the major known benefits.

The Stabilized Immune Modulating Components:

   x   Provide much of the language of *The Code of Life* for cellular recognition, intracellular communication, and communication between cells (intercellular) and the immune system.

   x   Contain antioxidant and free radical scavengers. The importance of antioxidants to overall health and longevity is profound. Not only do antioxidants protect us from tissue damaging free radicals such as protection of the skin from sun damage, the lungs from air pollution and second hand smoke, the retina of the eye, and even the destruction of DNA. Research indicates that the amounts of antioxidants we consume are directly proportional to how long we will live and the *quality* of our lives.

x   Possess hypoglycemic and blood sugar normalizing functions in both Type 1 and Type 2 diabetics.

x   Contain an insulin-like growth factor that lowers the required

amount of insulin needed to maintain normal blood sugar levels.

x   Reduce the amount of insulin needed, thereby reducing cardiovascular risk factors and stress on the pancreas and likely increasing its useful life, overall improvement of the intake of nutrients through the cell membrane.

x   Are incorporated into the cell membranes throughout the body, enhancing the membranes effectiveness regarding a number of known functions.

x   Enhance the excretion of toxins from the cells by a process known as *exocytosis.*

x   Possess anti-inflammatory functions particularly effective in ulcerative colitis and arthritis, due at least in part to the specific inhibition of leukotriene B-4, a highly pro-inflammatory substance.

x   Are likely to reduce the incidence of cancer, stroke, and heart disease. This is due primarily to the scientifically established fact that chronic inflammation increases the incidence of these conditions.

x   Possess antiviral, antibacterial, and antifungal effects which are of particular interest especially today, linked to the increased incidence of antibiotic resistant strains of bacteria that are no longer responsive to treatment. (This further establishes *why* the ingestion of these Aloe–derived polymannans are so helpful in preventing, normalizing, and correcting so many digestive tract disorders, including, but not limited to, gastric ulcers, colitis, ulcerative colitis, diarrhea, leaky gut syndrome . . . all because of the antibacterial and antiviral actions of these long chain polysaccharides). The antifungal effects may be another mechanism helping to explain why the ingestion of the stabilized Aloe vera is so effective in lowering blood sugar. Antifungal drugs, although harmful in other areas, have been shown to reduce the risks of developing Type 2 diabetes.

x   Possess immune modulating and immune stimulating effects. Examples of enhanced immune functions by the ingestion of these very long chain polysaccharides are: stimulation of antibody production (by leukocytes) and an increase in the number of killer T-cells produced. This expresses the tremendous importance in these immune stimulating functions. The levels of antibody present in our blood directly affects our ability to destroy pathogenic (disease causing) organisms. The killer T-cells are among our first line of defense in destroying dangerous bacteria and viruses and may even protect us from those responsible for an array of cancers.

x   Enhance chemotaxis, the migration of immune cells to a site of injury or infection, thereby initiating the repair and healing response; promoting tissue growth and regeneration.

x   Protect the mucous membranes lining the respiratory, gastrointestinal, and genitourinary tracts resulting in an increased resistance to infections.

x   Help stop and prevent the damage and leakage of the intestinal wall, thereby alleviating the stress from the immune system.

We have witnessed impressive results in patients with Inflammatory Bowel Disease (IBD: Crohn's Disease and Ulcerative Colitis), Irritable Bowel Syndrome (IBS), Gastroesophageal Reflux Disease (GERD), Heartburn, Diverticulitis, Chronic Fatigue Syndrome (CFS), Gastric Ulcers, Constipation, Diarrhea, Allergies, Food Intolerances, Lactose Intolerance, and Malabsorption, to name a few.

From MIT's Technology Review, February, 2003, _"If you don't have glycosylation . . ._ (the enzymatic breakdown and building up of varied complex carbohydrates) Ed. **... _You don't have life._"**

Chapter 8

The Critical Nature of Proper Digestion and the Role of the Complex Carbohydrate

Digestion is the process which permits us to extract the essential nutrients from our foods. Digestion which occurs *within* the digestive tract will be referred to as *extracellular digestion.*

The process of digestion begins in the mouth with mastication (chewing), breaking down the food into smaller particles. The food is mixed with saliva (which is now called chyme). This initiates the digestion of starches into sugars, and then this mixture is transported into the stomach by swallowing. In the stomach there are two very important functions that must occur. The first is that hydrochloric acid produced by the *chief cells* of the stomach is added to the chyme. This highly acidic condition is created for the breakdown of proteins to amino acids by a process known as hydrolysis. The second action is the addition of intrinsic factor (a glycoprotein) produced by the parietal cells of the stomach. Intrinsic factor is essential for the absorption of vitamin B-12. Poor absorption of vitamin B-12 causes anemia and in its most severe form is known as pernicious anemia, which is in some cases an autoimmune disease.

Without sufficient hydrochloric acid for the breakdown of proteins into amino acids, the absorption of these important nutrients will be prevented and the partially digested proteins will subsequently be available for the benefit of the pathogenic (disease causing) bacteria in the intestines. These harmful bacteria will then flourish, multiply, and produce their exotoxins which act as irritants causing diarrhea and/or irritable bowel syndrome, colitis, ulcerative colitis, etc. These toxins are then absorbed into our system placing an additional burden on the liver and kidneys which must process and eliminate them. Toxins suppress immune, metabolic, and organ function as well. Toxins are anti-enzymes. Enzymes are responsible for energy production, the breakdown and building up of nutrients and tissues, digestive and immune functions.

Many cases of indigestion are actually caused by a lack of stomach acid – not by too much! Additionally, lack of sufficient stomach acid is a cause of constipation which may be a causative factor in colon cancer. There is a study by Jeffery Bland, PhD, of the Linus Pauling Research Institute, that determined the beneficial effects of these Aloe healing components on the digestive process including regulation of gastrointestinal pH (acid-base balance) and the improvement of bowel regularity, improved gastrointestinal motility *"enhancement of energy and a greater sense of wellbeing."* There is also a decrease of pathogenic microorganisms and toxins in those participants.

The ingestion of these healing components has beneficial effects on gastric ulcers as well as the duodenum. They have protective as well as therapeutic effects due to the heavy layer of mucous containing mucopolysaccharides which coats the duodenum.

In the small intestine, pancreatic enzymes are added which further advance the digestion of carbohydrates, proteins, and fats. Bile is added from the gall bladder for the stimulation of peristalsis (propels contents through the intestine) and for the absorption of fat soluble vitamins such as vitamins D, A and K. Vitamin D has recently been shown to decrease the incidence of breast and colon cancer, as well as its known effect of preventing rickets and osteoporosis. Vitamin A supports immune function and is essential for sight. Vitamin K which is essential for blood clotting can be derived from the healthy or friendly bacteria that are supported by components found within these healing components. Throughout this extracellular digestive process, the chyme must move through the gastrointestinal tract at a certain rate called the *transmit time.* It should not be too fast as in diarrhea, so as to not afford the body the time it needs to absorb nutrients and not too slow, as in constipation, so as to cause putrefaction (build-up of disease causing bacteria, yeasts, and other pathogens and their toxic waste products). Numerous studies substantiate the normalization of digestive tract function with the ingestion of these Aloe healing components.

The Protectors

The cell does not want to be invaded by viruses, harmful bacteria, toxins, or any other foreign substance that would be detrimental. Fortunately, the cell can be protected by these complex carbohydrate polysaccharides known as mucopolysaccharides.

These essential complex carbohydrates also form a mucopolysaccharide coating on the surface of epithelial tissues throughout the body such as the mucous lining of the nasal passages, lungs, digestive, and genitourinary tracts. They are responsible for the protection of these structures and in part, explain why the ingestion of these complex carbohydrate mucopolysaccharides aid in the healing of gastric ulcers, GERD (Gastro Esophageal Reflux Disease), IBD (Irritable Bowel Syndrome), colitis, ulcerative colitis, Crohn's disease, and "Leaky Gut Syndrome" among others.

A review of some of the characteristics of these active healing components explains why they are effective in such a wide variety of digestive tract disorders. It is because of their many therapeutic properties including: anti-inflammatory, wound healing, pain relieving, immune boosting, pathogen killing, hydration retaining, and acid-base balancing effects. According to Dr. Lawrence G. Plaskett, B.A., Ph.D., C. Chem., F.R.I.C., *"Trials indicate... healing of peptic ulcers (stomach ulcers), controls intestinal secretions to normal levels, influences the bowel flora (microorganisms), controls gastric and intestinal pH (acid-base balance), improves the functioning of the pancreas, and limits adverse action in the colon reducing putrefaction."*

It is necessary for the stomach to produce both hydrochloric acid as well as pepsin, a protein digestive enzyme. It is interesting to note that many persons suffering from stomach pain, bloating, and indigestion will take antacids, often by the advice of their doctors. This may be ill advised due to the fact that there are many cases of alkaline indigestion where there is *insufficient* stomach acid, particularly in the elderly or persons with low blood pressure. If the stomach acid is reduced too much, bacterial growth will not be inhibited and gas will build up thereby creating acid reflux, GERD, and bloating. There is a pH balancing effect of the polymannans, which increases gastrointestinal pH, but to a much lesser degree, (0.45 vs. 2.55), compared to antacids, thereby permitting the breakdown of proteins in the stomach and at the same time eliminating ulcer pain. This applies equally to someone over-secreting stomach acid, as the polymannans will moderate the excess acid, and not reduce it to the point of stopping digestion. The completely non-toxic polymannans are also beneficial for the treatment of ulcers due to their tissue healing, analgesic, anti-inflammatory, and regenerating properties.

More scientific support for the therapeutic effects of the Aloe-derived polymannans comes from a paper written by Dr. Jeffrey Bland, at the Linus Pauling Institute of Science & Medicine in Palo Alto, California. The paper was published in *Preventive Medicine* in the March/April issue, 1985. In this paper Dr. Bland describes the following improvements in persons consuming the polmannans for one week: There was a 40% reduction in the Indican levels (a measure of intestinal putrefaction), there was an average reduction in specific gravity of the stools by 0.37 units (towards a more ideal value), and an improved composition of the beneficial bacterial flora. The yeast count was reduced markedly as well. This was interpreted to indicate better water-holding capacity of the stools as well as an improved transit time. This is of particular benefit because abnormally slow transit time (constipation) and abnormally rapid transportation time (diarrhea) are both harmful and indicative of abnormal function and the predisposition for other diseases such as *colon cancer* or *malabsorption syndromes.*

The Communicators

Complex carbohydrates carry specific recognition signals which identify themselves, and when attached to cell membranes, identify the cells to which they are attached. They are responsible for cell to cell communication and determine immunological recognition. These functions are of tremendous importance because such functions as recognition of (self from foreign), allergic, auto-immune diseases, and even the destruction of cancer cells are determined by the immune system's recognition and appropriate response to these identifying signals. We must emphasize that it is the carbohydrate molecules at the ends of these complex molecules that are responsible for this cellular identity.

Metaphorically speaking, the cell demands (orders) specific essential compounds and nutrients in order to perform its functions, repair itself, and to reproduce efficiently. Without the polysaccharides we do not have the *"order form"* and we do not have *"the order."* Without the polysaccharides, we do not have a language of communication to order, or fill the order.

In simple terms, the cell has sent a special order via *The Code of Life* to the enterocyte, specifying precisely what the cell requires. If these complex carbohydrate molecules are present in sufficient quantity, the order can be delivered into the interior of the cell.

In addition, as we touched upon previously, the enterocyte itself is protected by the mucopolysaccharide rich glycocalyx which covers these cells. The glycocalyx protects the cell, identifies the cell, and tells other cells what it requires nutritionally. It is essential for the mechanism of intracellular communication. As previously discussed, the cells are coated by this glycocalyx, sometimes referred to as *"the fuzz."* The fuzz is the polysaccharide matrix which identifies most cells throughout the body. It also contains these specific and non-specific receptor sites. This matrix is a significant part of *The Code of Life*. Without this polysaccharide matrix, cells could not communicate with one another and the essential functions of endocytosis (nutrition) and cellular recognition (immunity) would not occur.

The Miracle of Endocytosis

The significance of endocytosis cannot be overemphasized. The human body has a separate process distinct from the ordinary digestive process which enables the cells to take in these essential healing complex carbohydrates and other large macromolecules which have been shown to have a vast array of essential nutritional, developmental, and therapeutic effects.

Once these polymannans of varying chain lengths have been attached to the receptor site of the enterocyte, the receptor site creates an opening into the inside of the small intestine capable of ingesting these essential nutrients intact. They are then engulfed within the plasma membrane forming a coated vesicle. There is now formed within the enterocyte a coated vesicle which contains the ingested material. From there the coated vesicle is transported to the enterocyte cell wall, across the cell membrane and into the lymphatic system and finally into the bloodstream for distribution to hungry cells throughout the body.

Without the process of endocytosis we could not benefit from the intracellular utilization of these essential nutrients. This form of digestion takes place *within* the cell, the basic unit of life. These complex organic compounds are either utilized for their direct healing properties or are broken down within the cell by intracellular digestion.

Like extracellular digestion, *intracellular digestion* is another process which permits us to derive the essential nutrients from our diet. It supports *metabolism* whereby a biological entity processes a substance in order to mechanically and chemically convert the substance for the body to use. Metabolism is the complete set of chemical reactions that occur in living cells. *These metabolic processes are the basis of life as they allow cells to maintain their structures, respond to their environments, grow and reproduce.* Metabolism has two distinct divisions: *catabolism,* in which a cell breaks down complex molecules and tissues to yield energy and *anabolism,* in which a cell uses this energy to construct complex molecules, grow, repair, and perform its functions. Catabolism is the metabolic process that breaks down molecules into smaller units. Large polymeric molecules (polysaccharides, fatty acids, nucleic acids, and proteins) are processed into their constituent monomeric units (i.e., monosaccharides, carbon units, nucleotides, and amino acids respectively).

Anabolism is the metabolic process that builds larger molecules from smaller ones. Anabolic processes trend toward "building up" organs and tissues. These processes produce growth and differentiation of cells and increase in body size, a process that involves synthesis of complex molecules. Examples of anabolic processes include growth, tissue repair, replacement mineralization of bone, and increase of muscle mass.

Catabolism is the process of breaking down complex compounds into their basic constituents so that the body, through the process of anabolism, can then recombine them into new cells or tissues which arc necessary or needed. These components are *"the symbols"* that make up *The Code of Life.* It is the sum total of these communication processes that are responsible for repair, regeneration, growth, reproduction, a long and healthy life, and good health in general.

Intracellular digestion is facilitated by intracellular enzymes which can break down these complex compounds so that they can be built up into new cells and tissues as needed for growth, repair, and replacement. For this intracellular digestion to occur, certain essential nutrients must be provided to the cells that are not absorbed through the ordinary process of digestion, but through the fascinating process known as endocytosis.

Probiotics and the Polysaccharides

Your health is dependent not only on what you eat, but what you are able to digest. Digestion is key to preventing and curing diseases.

The digestive tract contains vast colonies of microorganisms collectively known as gut flora. These microorganisms or "bacteria" are of both the friendly and non-friendly types. The friendly bacteria perform many beneficial functions including the control of the pathogenic (disease causing), or "non-friendly" bacteria, which are known to produce toxins. A healthy balance must exist in favor of the friendly bacteria for optimum health.

This delicate balance may be adversely affected by disease, the use of excess alcohol, antibiotics, drugs, or other toxic substances and exposure to stress. In many cases these circumstances cause the beneficial friendly bacteria to decrease in number allowing the pathogenic disease-causing organisms to thrive to the detriment of our health. This is a prime example of environment or terrain change allowing pathogens to take hold. As discussed, pathogens are always present.

Maintenance of a healthy gut flora is, however, dependent on many factors, especially the quality of food intake. As mentioned elsewhere in this book, the immune modulators have been demonstrated to improve the microbial content of the digestive tract, thereby helping to maintain a healthy balance of organisms which aids in healing damaged tissues.

We must understand that every nutritional supplement we ingest and every bite of food we swallow, no matter what its level of nutritional quality, can be of much greater benefit to our body provided that the digestion capabilities are operating at an optimum.

The role of the immune modulators with their many healing properties, also improve digestion, optimizing the nutritional absorption from our foods and supplements.

The list of profound statements and conclusions published by researchers concerning the healing components discussed in this book would fill many volumes. We have published a few here to give the reader a flavor for the gravity of these conclusions to date.

H. Reginald McDaniel, M.D. states: *"The use of Aloe vera will be the most important single step forward in the treatment of disease in the history of mankind." By the ingestion of the Aloe-derived polymannans we can help to maintain a more active, vigilant, and powerful immune system."*

Dr. John C. Pitmann, M.D., states: *"The key to integrating healthy digestion with a healthy immune system is the oral ingestion of Aloe mucilaginous polysaccharides."* He also states: *"Aloe mucilaginous polysaccharides act as a potent anti-inflammatory agent, stopping the damage and leakage of the intestinal wall, thereby taking the stress off the immune system."...* *"Aloe mucilaginous polysaccharides stimulate the macrophages, monocytes, antibodies, and T-cells. Phagocytosis (the process of white blood cells engulfing bacteria, viruses, etc.) is dramatically increased to ingest foreign proteins such as the HIV virus."...* *"Aloe mucilaginous polysaccharides increase the number and intensity of all immune cells in the body."...* *"Aloe mucilaginous polysaccharides have direct anti-bacterial, anti-viral, antifungal/yeast and anti-parasite effects. Chronic yeast growth can be controlled so the normal, healthy flora (friendly bacteria Ed.) can then thrive more easily."*

..."Aloe mucilaginous polysaccharides have a remarkable ability to normalize an array of damaging processes, which has the effect of enhancing the immune system function through improved digestion."

Ivan Danhoff, M.D., PhD, states: *"Aloe mucilaginous polysaccharide molecules cause the body to produce a natural chemical, tumor necrosis factor, which functions to shut off the blood supply to tumors."...* *"Aloe mucilaginous polysaccharides are immune modulating, which have a powerful healing effect on many different immune system disorders."...* *"Aloe mucilaginous polysaccharides have a direct anti-bacterial and ant-viral effect."...* *"Where as vitamins and minerals can only function outside the cells, mucilaginous polysaccharides are very effective intracellular antioxidants and free radical scavengers."...* *"Aloe mucilaginous polysaccharides ARE NOT DIGESTED by the enzyme systems in the human digestive tract; the mannose containing molecules are absorbed by endocytosis, i.e., THEY ARE TAKEN UP INTO THE CELL INTACT."* *"These very large long beads, these very long necklaces* (long-chain Aloe polymannans) Ed., *have a profound effect in preventing disease and protecting us from various noxious agents in the environment."*

Dr. Lawrence Plaskett, B.A., Ph.D., C. Chem., F.R.S.C. states": *"It will be clear why Aloe is dubbed with emotive terms such as "The Silent Healer" and even "Panacea." This happens even among quite well informed users of Aloe, not just people who are easily influenced by hype and imagination. It does so because the nature of the fundamental actions of Aloe are to improve the status of some vitally important systems in the body which affect many functions."*

"Aloe greatly enhances the efforts of the practioners to support the patients immune system, to promote healing, and to cleanse and relieve inflammatory conditions."..."The healing action of Aloe depends partly upon the direct stimulatory effect upon the fibroblasts and other cell types and partly upon the consequences of the tissues being better cleanse" (detoxified, Ed.).

"Trials indicate that Aloe vera heals peptic ulcers, controls intestinal secretions to normal levels, influences the bowel flora, controls gastric and intestinal pH, improves the functioning of the pancreas, and limits adverse bacteria action in the colon, reducing putrefaction."

"The most marked biological activities of mannans in mammals are activation of macrophages and stimulation of T lymphocytes." Ian R. Tizard, BVMS, Ph.D., Robert H. Carpenter, CVM, MS, Bill H. McAnalley, Ph.D. and Maurice C. Kemp, Ph.D.

Dr. Terry Pulse states: *"If you can hold the process of disease in check, and if you can stimulate and enhance one's own defense mechanism, which is your immune system, there are no conditions that your body is not capable of conquering and Aloe vera is one of those principles."*

Conclusion

Our bodies have not changed to any significant degree over the last century, yet our foods have become depleted in vital phytonutrients, and in particular the vital immune modulating components.

As previously discussed, the lack of these components is the basis for C.I.C.D.S. (Cellular and Immune Communication Deficiency Syndrome), which opens the door for autoimmunity diseases and pre-mature aging. (See Chapter 4, "What has happened to our food?").

If we do not receive the essential nutrients our bodies require, we are more susceptible to disease of all types. Simple stated, C.I.C.D.S. is the inevitable outcome due to the lack of vital and specific nutrients. Because of this unavoidable fact, it may be accurately stated that the overwhelming majority of humans on the planet currently suffer from C.I.C.D.S. to many varying degrees.

C.I.C.D.S. creates an environment which could be characterized as an open door to an endless list of degenerative diseases and disorders. With diseases rising at the alarming rates now being documented, it is more than apparent that the majority of us are increasingly susceptible.

Health, strength, youth, beauty, prevention and recovery from disease begin at the cellular level. Nutrition is not just about "what you eat." It is mainly about what you are capable of digesting, and subsequently; what is ultimately delivered into your cells.

Maintaining a healthy internal environment is the basis of prevention, health, anti-aging and longevity.

With adequate consumption of immune modulating components and phytonutrients, you may expect the following:

•   An array of system support will occur throughout your entire body.

•   First and foremost, you will be restoring digestive function enabling any subsequent nutrient you ingest to enter your blood stream, and ultimately all thirteen trillion of your cells, and cell nucleuses, the home of your DNA.

•   You will be providing your cells with unmatched vital nourishment and support. With the building blocks of cellular communication through The Code of Life, your cells will progressively be able to perform their physiological functions as designed. This cellular recognition and communication is so vitally important for proper immune function, the recognition of self versus foreign cells, and subsequently the elimination of autoimmunity, the driving force behind eighty-five percent of the chronic diseases known to man.

•   The immune modulating components will enable your digestive tract to establish a healthier environment by reducing the number of disease-causing bacteria, viruses, fungi, and parasites while enhancing the growth of the friendly bacteria.

•   As the modulators begin the healing processes in your digestive tract, digestive diseases, symptoms, and deficiencies begin to dissipate. Dissipating diseases and their dissipating symptoms are soon to follow as the modulators are utilized by all systems, organs and cells.

•   In your blood, the effects of enhanced immune function will begin to occur as the production of your disease fighting white blood cells increase. The enhancement of chemotaxis and wound healing will be progressively promoted.

•   Improvements in blood sugar levels, vital for diabetics and essential for the maintenance of your metabolism, brain, and organ function occur naturally over time.

•   Your body begins to receive the cardiovascular benefits of the reduction of   elevated   cholesterol   and   triglycerides. Anti-inflammatory effects reduce pain and swelling in every area of the body.

•   Antioxidant   effects   inactivate   free   radicals   and   slow premature aging. Immune modulating components and bio-active phytonutrients in general provide many of the essential building blocks for so many tissues throughout your body such as heparin which prevents abnormal blood clotting, glucosamine, a component of healthy cartilage, enhanced   collagen   formation   for beautiful healthy skin, healthy bones, ligaments, tendons, muscles, skin, connective tissues, the myelin sheath which covers and protects nerves, hyaluronic acid, essential for fertilization and a component of the intervertebral discs of your spine, and the identity and recognition of your blood and tissue types. As discussed, the list is virtually endless.

The discovery of this phenomenon and the understanding of how phytonutrients, and in particular the complex carbohydrates, promote health and youth at the cellular level is the single most important advancement in healing, preventative medicine, and anti-aging ever discovered. It is this discovery that has immediately threatened the current "health-care" monopoly of the pharmaceutical industry.

Now that you understand why this life-saving information is not being emphasized to the public by main-stream sources. It has now become your responsibility as well to spread this wonderful news. Big Pharma will be continuing to do doing everything in their power to block and suppress the knowledge of The Code. The elimination of The Plague and The Cartel's big business with disease is dependent upon one hope. How quickly can we, together, spread this life-saving information worldwide?

Potentially Save or Extend a Life Today!

Send a copy of *The Code of Life...* to a friend or loved one.

They will appreciate it!!

<u>DrRonPDrucker.com</u>

Below is the original oath and doctrine designed as a moral, professional and ethical standard for the medical profession:

THE HIPPOCRATIC OATH

I swear by Apollo the physician, by Æsculapius, Hygeia, and Panacea, and I take to witness all the gods, all the goddesses, to keep according to my ability and my judgment, the following Oath.

"To consider dear to me as my parents him who taught me this art; to live in common with him and if necessary to share my goods with him; to look upon his children as my own brothers, to teach them this art if they so desire without fee or written promise; to impart to my sons and the sons of the master who taught me and the disciples who have enrolled themselves and have agreed to the rules of the profession, but to these alone the precepts and the instruction. **I will prescribe regimen for the good of my patients according to my ability and my judgment and never do harm to anyone. To please no one will I prescribe a deadly drug nor give advice which may cause his death.** Nor will I give a woman a pessary to procure abortion. But I will preserve the purity of my life and my art. I will not cut for stone, even for patients in whom the disease is manifest; I will leave this operation to be performed by practitioners, specialists in this art. In every house where I come I will enter only for the good of my patients, keeping myself far from all intentional ill-doing and all seduction and especially from the pleasures of love with women or with men, be they free or slaves. **All that may come to my knowledge in the exercise of my profession or in daily commerce with men, which ought not to be spread abroad, I will keep secret and will never reveal.** If I keep this oath faithfully, may I enjoy my life and practice my art, respected by all men and in all times; but if I swerve from it or violate it, may the reverse be my lot."

We can clearly see that the pledges within the first and second bolded sentences have been all but cast into obscurity. Could the heads of the medical and pharmaceutical industries be grossly misconstruing the meaning and purpose of the third bolded sentence?

References

Research for *The Code of Life...* includes:

20 Freeze, H. Disorders in protein glycosylation and potential therapy: Tip of an iceberg? J. Pediatrics. 1998; 133 (5): 595-600.

A Chemical Investigation of Aloe Barbadensis Miller; G.R. Waller, S. Mangiafico & C.R. Ritchey.

A Clinical Pilot Study Using Carrisyn in the Treatment of Acquired Immunodeficiency Syndrome (AIDS); H. Reg McDaniel, Sue Perkins & B.H. McAnalley.

A Comparative Investigation of Methods Used to Estimate Aloin & Related Compounds in Aloes.

A Drug for all Seasons Medical and Pharmacological History of Aloe; John S. Haller, Jr., Ph.D.

A Mucilage from Aloe Vera; Elizabeth Roboz & A.J. Haagen-Smit, Shu XO and others.

A population-based case-control study of childhood leukemia in Shanghai. Cancer 1988 Aug 1; 62(3):635-44.

A Phytochemical Study of Aloe Vera Leaf; Tom D. Rowe & Lloyd M. Parks.

AIDS and the Immune System; Warner C. Greene.

ASA, Aloe Vera Rx vs. Frostbite; Charlene Laino.

Acute Oral Toxicity Study (Dawson Research Corporation).

Acute Oral Toxicity Study of Aloe vera Powder in Rats (Dawson Research Corporation).

Advances in the Immunobiology of the Skin. Implications for Cutaneous Malignancies; Margaret L. Kripke & Cynthia A. Romerdahl.

Allergy and the Immune System; Lawrence M. Lichtenstein.

Aloctin A, an Active Substance of Aloe Arborescens Miller as an Immunomodulator; Ken'ichi Imanishi.

Aloe and Other Topical Antibacterial Agents in Wound Healing (Aloe Today, Fall/Winter 1993); John P. Heggers, Ph.D.

Aloe as an Ingredient; J.A. Magnuson.

Aloe Barbadensis Extracts Reduce the Production of Interleukin-10 After Exposure to Ultraviolet Radiation; Ronald P. Pelley, Ph.D., M.D.

Aloe Can Rise to the Challenge (Article for Aloe Today – Ronald P. Pelley, Ph.D., M.D.)

Aloe Drug May Mimic AZT Without Toxicity, Medical World News, December 1987 issue, Dr. H. Reginald McDaniel.

Aloe Medicinal Substances; Dr. Wendell Winters.

Aloe Polysaccharides and Their Measurement; Ronald P. Pelley, Ph.D., M.D.

Aloe species have been reported to have several biological activities, including: immunomodulation Suzuki, et al., 1979; Yoshimoto et al., 1987; Winters et al., 1981; Yagi et al, 1985; and Saito, 1993, enhancement of wound healing (Heggars, et al., 1993) and antiinflammatory actions (Davis et al., 1989).

Aloe Vera; Alexander G. Schauss.

Aloe Vera; Alan D. Klein & Neal S. Penneys.

Aloe Vera (Aloe Barbadensis Miller); Ivan E. Danhof, Ph.D., M.D.

Aloe Vera, Alan D. Klein, M.D., and Neal S. Penneys, M.D., Ph.D. Miami, FL; Journal of the American Academy of Dermatology. Volume 18, Number 4, Part I, pgs. 714-720, April 1988.

Aloe Vera – A Natural Approach for Treating Wounds, Edema, and Pain in Diabetes; Robert H. Davis, Ph.D., Mark G. Leitner, Joseph M. Russo.

Aloe Vera and Burn Wound Healing; Teddy Kaufman, A.R. Newman & M.R. Wexler.

Aloe Vera – Aloe Vera and Cancer, Dr. Lawrence G. Plaskett, B.A., Ph.D., C. Chem., F.R.I.C., Aloe Vera Information Service, Issue 6, Biomedical Information Services, Ltd., Cornwall.

Aloe Vera and Gibberellin Anti-Inflammatory Activity in Diabetes; Robert H. Davis, Ph.D. & Nicholas P. Maro.

Aloe Vera – Aloe Vera and the Four A's Arthritis, Atheroma, Angina and Asthma, Dr. Lawrence G. Plaskett, B.A., Ph.D., C. Chem., F.R.I.C., Aloe Vera Information Service, Issue 15, Biomedical Information Services, Ltd., Cornwall.

Aloe Vera – Aloe and its Quality Control – Checking upon the Genuineness of Products, Dr. Lawrence G. Plaskett, B.A., Ph.D., C. Chem., F.R.I.C., Aloe Vera Information Service, Issue 11, Biomedical Information Services, Ltd., Cornwall.

Aloe Vera: Aloe Vera and Cancer, Aloe Vera and the Human Immune System, Aloe Vera and the Human Digestive System, Aloe Eases Inflammation, The Healing Properties of Aloe Vera, Aloe Vera: Aloe Vera in Alternative Medicine Practice, Aloe Eases Inflammation, Dr. G. Lawrence Plaskett.

Aloe Vera and Inflammation; Robert H. Davis, Joseph M. Kabbani & Nicholas P. Maro.

Aloe Vera and Wound Healing; Robert H. Davis, Joseph M. Kabbani & Nicholas P. Maro.

Aloe Vera Anti-Viral Agent; Ruth Adams.

Aloe Vera – The Carbohydrate Fraction of Aloe, Dr. Lawrence G. Plaskett, B.A., Ph.D., C. Chem., F.R.I.C., Aloe Vera Information Service, Issue 12, Biomedical Information Services, Ltd., Cornwall.

Aloe Vera and the Human Immune System, Dr. Lawrence Plaskett, B.A., Ph.D., C. Chem., F.R.S.C., The Aloe Vera Information Service, Issue I.

Aloe Vera and the Inflamed Synovial Pouch Model; Robert H. Davis, Greta J. Stewart, Peter J. Bregman.

Aloe vera (Aloe Barbadensis Miller), Internal Uses of Aloe Vera, Potential Benefits from Orally-Ingested Internal Aloe Vera Gel, Ivan E. Danhof, Ph.D, M.D.

Aloe Vera and the Human Digestive System, Lawrence Plaskett, B.A., Ph.D., C. Chem., F.R.S.C., Biomedical Information Services, Ltd., Cornwall.

Aloe Vera and the Human Digestive System, Aloe Eases Inflammation and Aloc Vera in Alternative Medicine; Lawrence Plaskett B.A., Ph.D., C. Chem., F.R.S.C.

Aloe Vera: Fact or Quakery; David C. Spoerke & Brent R. Ekins.

Aloe Vera For Burns; William F. Kivett, M.D.

Aloe Vera Gel and its Effect on Cell Growth; William B. Bowles.

Aloe Vera Gel: What is the Evidence? Judith M. Marshall.

Aloe Vera Gel in Peptic Ulcer Therapy: Preliminary Report Julian J. Blitz, D.O., James W. Smith, D.O. & Jack R. Gerardo, D.O., Dania, Florida; Journal of the American Osteopathic Association, Vol. 62, April 1963.

Aloe Vera Goes Maquila; Tony Vindell.

Aloe Vera, Hydrocortisone, and Sterol Influence on Wound Tensile Strengh and Anti-Inflammation; Robert H. Davis, Ph.D., Joseph J. Di Donato, B.S., Richard W.S. Johnson, Christopher B. Stewart.

Aloe Vera in the Treatment of Roentgen Ulcers & Telangiectasis; Carroll S. Wright. M.D.

Aloe Vera: Internal & External First Aid.

Aloe Vera is a Good Vehicle for Estrogens; Robert H. Davis, Ph.D., Joseph J. Di Donato, B.S.

Aloe Vera – It's Chemical and Therapeutic Properties, Ronald M. Shelton, MAJ, USAF, MC; International Journal of Dermatology, October 1991.
Aloe Vera Open Wound Healing Micro-Assay; Robert H. Davis, Ph.D., Joseph J. Di Donato, B.S.

Aloe Vera Produces Anti-Inflammatory, Immune Strengthening Effects on Skin; Steven R. Schechter, N.D.

Aloe Vera Revered, Mysterious Healer (Health Food Business Magazine – Timothy R. Fox).

Aloe Vera, Salicylic Acid & Aspirin for Burns; Azriel Frumkin, M.D.

Aloe Vera: The Healing Plant, Stephen R. Schecter, N.D.

Aloe Vera the Miraculous Healer Lee Cowden, M.D. Health Consciousness, 1992, Vol. 13, No. 1, pp. 25. John C. Pittman, MD. Health Consciousness, 1992, Volume 13, No. 1, pp. 28-30.

Aloe Vera Rio Grande Valley Folks Claim It's Good for What Ails You (Texas Highways Magazine).

Aloe Vera: Witchcraft or Wonder Drug? Martha A. Walton.

Aloe Versatile (Fort Worth Star Telegram).

Aloe's effectiveness As an Antiinflammatory Agent Dr. Hiroko Saito, Dept. of pharmacy, Aichi Cancer Center, Nagoya, Japan. Aloe Today, Spring 1993.

Aloes in the Treatment of Burns and Scalds, J.E. Crewe, Md., Rochester, Minnesota.

Aloes of the World: A Checklist, Index and Code; Trevor B.D. Harding.

Amazing Aloe – This desert plant heals skin and much more, Karen France Unruh, Reprint: Tanning Trends, May 1989.

American Journal of Clinical Nutrition, 40 (4 Suppl): 927-30, Oct., 1984.Nair, P., et al.

"Amino acid metabolism in pediatric patients" Nutrition 14 (1): 143-8, Imura K., Okada A (1998).

An Anti-Complementary Polysaccharide with Immunological Adjuvant Activity from the Leaf Parenchyma Gel of Aloe Vera; L.A. 'T Hart, A.J.J. Van Den Berg, L. Kuis, H. Van Dijk & R.P. Labadie.

Ancient Herb in New Form Delivers Proven Effects; Keisuke Fujita, M.D., Ph.D., Hidenhiko Beppu, Ph.D., Kaoru Kawai, Ph.D. & Kan Shinpo, Ph.D.

Angiogenesis inhibited by drinking tea. Nature. 1999; 398:381Cao Y, Cao R.

Anthraquinone Derivatives in Vegetable Laxatives; F.H.L. van Os.

Antibradykinin Active Material in Aloe Saponaria; Akira Yagi, Nobuo Harada, Hidenori Yamada, Shuichi Iwadare & Itsuo Nishioka.

Antidiabetic Activity of Aloe Vera Juice. Clinical Trial in New cases Of Diabetes mellitus; S. Yongchaiyudha, V. Rungpitarangsi, N. Bunyapraphtsara & O. Chokechaijaroenporn.

Antidiabetic activity of Aloe Vera L.Juice II. Clinical trial in new cases of diabetes mellitus, S. Yongchaiyudha, V. Rungpitarangsi, N. Bunyapraphatsara, and O. Chokechaijaroenporn; Phytomedicine Vol. 3(3), pp. 241-243, 1996: 1996 by Gustav Fischer Verlag, Stuttgart-Jen-New York.

Anti-inflammatory Activity and Wound Healing Activity of a Growth Substance in Aloe Vera, Anti-inflammatory Activity of Aloe Vera against a Spectrum of Irritants, Aloe Vera and Inflammation, The Conductor Orchestrator Concept of Aloe Vera, Aloe Vera Open Wound Healing Micro-Assay, Robert H. Davis, Ph.D, Joseph J. Di Donato, Glenn M. Hartman, Richard C. Haas.

Anti-inflammatory Activity of Aloe Vera Against A Spectrum of Irritants; Robert H. Davis, Ph.D., Mark G. Leitner, Joseph M. Russo, Megan E. Byrne.

Anti-inflammatory activity of extracts from Aloe vera gel; Beatriz Vazquez a, Guillermo Avila a, David Segura a, Bruno Escalante b Journal Ethnopharmacology 55 (1996) 69-75.

Anti-Inflammatory, Analgesic and Wound Healing Activity of Aloe Vera; Robert H. Davis, Ph.D.

Anti-inflammatory & Wound Healing Properties of Aloe Vera, Dr. Wendell Winters, et al.

Antioxidant defense systems: the role of carotenoids, tocopherols, and thiols. Am. J. Clin. Nutr., 53:194S-200S; Di Mascio, P., M. E. Murphy, and H. Sies. (1991).

Antioxidant properties of (-)-epicatechin-3-gallate and its inhibition of Cr (VI)-induced DNA damage and Cr (IV)- or TPA-stimulated NF-Kappa B activation. Mol Cell Biochem. 2000; 206:125-132; Shi X, Ye J, Leonard SS, et al.

Antioxidants Winning the Fight for Good Health; Frank Murray.

Antioxidative Substances in Leaves of Polygonum Hydropiper; Hiroyuki Haraguchi, Kensuke Hashimoto & Akira Yagi.

Antithrombotic activities of green tea catechins and (-)-epigallocatechin gallate. Throm Res. 1999; 96:229-237; Kang WS, Lim IH, Yuk DY, et al.

Antiviral Activity of Aloe Extracts Against Cytomegalovirus; Dr. Wendell Winters.

Autoimmune Diseases; Lawrence Steinman.

Bacteriostatic Property of Aloe Vera; Lorna J. Lorenzetti, Rupert Salisbury, Jack Beal & Jack N. Baldwin.

Basis of Aloe Certification; Yin-Tung Wang, Ph.D.

Beneficial Effect of Aloe on Wound Healing in an Excisional Wound Model; Dr. Wendell Winters.

Beneficial Effects of Aloe in Wound Healing; John P. Heggers, Ronald P. Pelly & Martin C. Robson.

Beneficial Effects of Aloe on Wound Healing in an Excisional Wound Model; John P. Heggers, Ahmet Kucukcelebi, Dimitri Listengarten.

Beta-sitosterol, a plant sterol, induces apoptosis and activates key caspases in MDA-MB-231 human breast cancer cells. Oncol Rep. 2003; 10(2):497-500. (PubMed); Awad AB, Roy R, Fink CS.

Beta-sitosterol activates the sphingomyelin cycle and induces apoptosis in NCaP human prostate cancer cells. Nutr Cancer. 1998;32(1):8-12. (PubMed); von Holtz RL, Fink CS, Awad AB.

Biochemical Properties of Carboxypeptidase in Aloe Arborescens Miller Var. Natalensis Berger; Shosuke Ito, Ryo Teradaira, Hidehiko Beppu, Masafumi Obata & Keisuke Fujita.

BIOFLAVINOIDS AND POLYPHENOLS: MEDICAL APPLICATIONS. Brian E. Leibovitz, Ph.D and Jennifer Ann Mueller, B.S.

Biological Activity of Aloe Vera; R.H. Davis.

Biological Standardization of Aloe Vera; Robert H. Davis, Ph.D.

Biologically Active Constituents of Leaves and Roots of Aloe Arborescens var. Natalensis; Toshifumi Hirata & Takayuki Suga.

Botanical Science Helps to Develop a New Relief For Human Suffering; Claud L. Horn.

Bradykinin-Degrading Glycoprotein in Aloe Arborescens var. Natalensis; Akira Yagi, Nobou Harada, Koichiro Shimomura & Itsuo Nishioka.

Bradykinninase Activity of Aloe Extract; Keisuke Fujita, Ryoji Teradaira & Toshiharu Nagatsu, Keisuke Fujita, Yasuo Yamada, Keizou Azuma & Susumu Hirozawa.

Cancer-Fighting Foods (Harvard Health Letter).

Cancer prevention by carotenoids. Mutat. Res., 402:159-163; Nishino, H. (1998)

Cancer Study Finds Sunscreen is Poor Shields; Gautam Nalk.

Carbohydrate Polymers From Aloe Ferox Leaves; Wilfred T. Mabusela, Alistair M. Stephen & Marthinus C. Botha.

Carotenoids: an overview. Meth. Enzymol., 213: 3-13; Pfander, H. (1992).

Carotenoids and the immune response. J. Nutr., 119:112-115; Bendich, A. (1989).

Carotenoid content of fruits and vegetables: an evaluation of analytic data. J. Am. Diet. Assoc., 93:284-296; Mangels, A.R., J.M. Holden, G.R. Beecher, M.R. Forman, and E. Lanza. (1993).

Carotenoids today and challenges for the future. In: Britton, G., S. Liaaen-Jensen, and H. Pfander [eds], Carotenoids vol. 1A: Isolation and Analysis. Basel: Birkhäuser; Britton, G., S. Liaaen-Jensen, and H. Pfander. (1995).

Carrington Gets USDA Approval to Market Drug to Veterinarians (The Dallas Morning News – Joe Simnacher).

Changes in prostanoid synthesis in response to diet and hypertension in one-kidney, one clip rats. Hypertension 1985; 7:886-92; Codde JP, McGowan HM, Vandongen R, Beilin LJ.

Changes of blood pressure in spontaneously hypertensive rats dependent on the quantity and quality of fat intake. Biomed.Biochim.Acta 1985; 44:1491-505; Moritz V, Singer P, Forster D, Berger I, Massow S.

Changes of N-6 and N-3 fatty acids in spontaneously hypertensive (SHR) and normotensive rats after diets supplemented with alpha-linolenic or eicosapentaenoic acids. Prostaglandins Leukot.Med. 1987;28:183-93; Singer P, Berger I, Gerhard U, Wirth M, Moritz V, Forster D.

Characteristics of Polysaccharides of Aloe Barbadensis Miller: Part III-Structure of an Acidic Oligosaccharide; Gaurhai Mandal, Rina Ghosh & Amalendu Das.

Chemical Characterization of the immunomodulating polysaccaride of Aloe Vera L; Jimmy Tai-Nin Chow, David A. Williamson, Kenneth M. Yates, Warren J. Goux.

Chemical Studies of Aloe Vera Juice II; G.D. Bouchy & Gunnar Gjerstad.

"Clinical Severity and Thermodynamic Effects of Iron-Responsive Element Mutations in Hereditary Hyperferritinemia-Cataract Syndrome." Journal of Biological Chemistry 274 (1999): 26439–26447; Allerson, Charles R., M. Cazzola, and Tracey A. Rouault.

Comparative Studies of Aloe From Commercial Sources; Todd Waller.

Conformational Studies of Natural Products. III (*)Confomration of Natural 8-C-Glucosyl-7Hydroxy-5-Methylchromones & Their Derivatives (**); Paolo Manitto, Diego Monti & Giovanna Speranza.

Considerations for use of probiotic bacteria to modulate human health. J. Nutr. 2000: 130:384S-390S. Entrez PubMed 10721912, Sanders ME.

Current Status of Quality Control of Aloe Barbadensis Extracts; R.P. Pelley, Y.T. Wang & T.A. Waller.

Designing a Personal Care Product Using Aloe Vera; Todd Waller.

Determination of the Position of the O-Acetyle Group in a B-(1-----4_-Mannan (acemannan) from Aloe Barbadensis Miller; Sukumar Manna & Bill H. McAnalley.

Dietary antioxidant intake and risk of type 2 diabetes. DIABETES CARE (2): 362-366; Montonen J, Knekt P, Jarvinen R, et al. (2004).

Dietary fat intake and risk of lung cancer: a prospective study of 51,452 Norwegian men and women. Eur J Cancer Prev 1997 Dec;6(6):540-9; Veierod MG, Laake P, Thelle DS.

Dietary fish oil normalize dyslipidemia and glucose intolerance with unchanged insulin levels in rats fed a high sucrosc diet. Biochim.Biophys.Acta 1996; 1299:175-82; Lombardo YB, Chicco A, D'Alessandro ME, Martinelli M, Soria A, Gutman R.

Dietary fish oil prevents dexamethasone induced hypertension in the rat. Clin Sci.(Lond) 1985;69:691-9; Codde JP, Beilin LJ.

Dietary fish oil reduces progression of chronic inflammatory lesions in a rat model of granulomatous colitis. Gut 1990; 31:539-44; Vilaseca J, Salas A, Guarner F, Rodriguez R, Martinez M, Malagelada JR.

Dietary manipulation in experimental inflammatory bowel disease. Agents Actions 1992; Spec No:C10-C14; Guarner F, Vilaseca J, Malagelada JR.

Different Effects of Native Candida Albicans Mannan & Mannan-Derived Oligosaccharides on Antigen-Stimulated Lymphoproliferation In Vitro; Raymond P. Podzorski, Gary R. Gray & Robert D. Nelson.

Does Aloe Vera Have Strogenic Activity? Robert H. Davis, Ph.D., Joseph J. Di Donato, B.S.

Effect of Aloe Barbedensis & Clofibrate on Serum Lipids in Triton-Induced Hyperlipidaemia in Presbytis Monkeys; V.P. Dixit & Suresh Joshi.

Effect of Aloe Extract on Peripheral Phagocytosis in Adult Bronchial Asthma, Takao Shida, Akira Yagi, Hiroshi Nishimura, and Itsuo Nishioka; Received: December 10, 1984; accepted: February 24, 1985; Planta Medica 1985.

Effect of Aloe Lectin on Deoxyribonucleic Acid Synthesis in Baby Hamster Kidney Cells; A. Yagi, K. Machii, H. Nishimura, T. Shida & I. Nishioka.

Effect of Amino Acids in Aloe Extract on Phagocytosis By Peripheral Neutrophil in Adult Bronchial Asthma, Akira Yagi.

Effect of Leaf Extracts of Aloe Arborescens Mill Subsp. Natalensis Berger on Growth of Trichophyton Metagrophytes; Keisuke Fujita, Ryoji Teradaira & Toshiharu Nagatsu, Keisuke Fujita, Yasuo Yamada, Keizou Azuma & Susumu Hirozawa.

Effect of long-term consumption of a probiotic bacterium, Lactobacillus rhamnosus GG, in milk on dental caries and caries risk in children. Caries Res. 2001; 35:412-20. Entrez PubMed 11799281, Nase L, Hatakka K, Savilahti E, Saxelin M, Ponka A, Poussa T, Korpela R, Meurman JH.

Effect of long term consumption of probiotic milk on infections in children attending day care centres: double blind, randomised tiral. BMJ. 2001; 322:1327. Entrez PubMed 11387176, Hatakka K, Savilahti E, Ponka A, Meurman JH, Poussa T, Nase L, Saxelin M, Korpela R.

Effect of moderate levels of dietary fish oil on insulin secretion and sensitivity, and pancreas insulin content in normal rats. Ann.Nutr Metab 1996; 40:61-70; Chicco A, D'Alessandro ME, Karabatas L, Gutman R, Lombardo YB.

Effect of Orally Consumed Aloe vera Juice on Gastrointestinal Function in Normal Humans Jeffrey Bland, PhD, Linus Pauling Insittute of Science & Medicine, Palo Alto, California.

Effect of Preservatives on Aloe Vera Mucilage; A.H. Ghanem, A.F. Shalaby & M. Helal.

Effect of UV Irradiation on Lethal Infection of Mice with Candida Albicans; Margate L. Kripke & Y.M. Denkins.

Effects of Aloe Extracts on Human Normal and Tumor Cells in Vitro and Immunoreactive Lectins in Leaf Gel from Aloe Barbadensis Miller "Physiotherapy research", Vol. 7, s23-s25 (1993) Wendell D. Winters W.D. Winters, R. Benevides, and W. J, Clouse Economic Botany, 35 (1), 1991, pp 89-95.

Effects of feeding various tocotrienol sources on plasma lipids and aortic atherosclerotic lesions in cholesterol-fed rabbits. FOOD RESEARCH INTERNATIONAL 35 (2-3): 245-251; Hasselwander O, Kramer K, Hoppe PP, et al. (2002).

Effects of Low Molecular Constituents from Aloe Vera Gel on Oxidative Metabolism and Cytotoxic and Bactericidal Activities of Human Neutrophils, L.A. T Hart, P.H. Nibbering, M.Th. Van Barselaar, H. van Dijk.

Effects of Ultraviolet-B Radiation on Human Health; Margaret L. Kripke, Dulloo AG, Duret C, Rohrer D, et al.

Efficacy of a green tea extract rich in catechin polyphenols and caffeine in increasing 24-h energy expenditure and fat oxidation in humans. Am J Clin Nutr. 1999; 70:1040-1045.

Enhancement of Aloe-Responsiveness of Human Lymphocytes by Acemmanan (Carrisyn); Debra Womble & J. Harold Helderman.

Enhancement of Two-Stage Skin Carcinogenesis by Exposure of Distant Skin to UV Radiation; Margaret L. Kripke, Paul T. Stickland & Donald Creasia.

Epigallocatechin gallate and gallocatechin gallate in green tea catechins inhibit extracellular release of Vero toxin from enterohemorrhagic Escherichia coli. O157:H7. Biochem Biophys Acta. 1999; 1472:42-50; Sugita-Konishi Y, Hara-Kudo Y, Amano F, et al.

Evaluation of Acemannan in the Treatment of Recurrent Aphthouse Stomatitis; Jacqueline M. Plemons, Terry D. Rees, William H. Binnie, John M. Wright, Ingrid Guo & John E. Hall.

Evidence for protection against age-related macular degeneration by carotenoids and antioxidant vitamins. Am. J. Clin. Nutr., 62(suppl):1448S-1461S; Snodderly, D.M. (1995).

Experimental Use of Aloe Vera Extract in Clinical Practice; Robert B. Northway, D.V.M.

Folk Uses and Commercial Exploitation of Aloe Leaf Pulp; Julia F. Morton.

Food Technology, 47: 85-90, April 1993; Kinsella, J.E., et al.

Frostbite – Methods to Minimize Tissue Loss; J.P. Heggers, Robert L. McCauley & Martin C. Robson.

Further Studies of the Glucomannan from Aloe Vahombe (Liliaceae). II. Partial Hydrolyses & NMR 13C Studies; Farhad Radjabi-Nassab, Christine Ramiliarison, Claude Monneret & Erna Vilkas.

Gamma-Tocotrienol metabolism and antiproliferative effect in prostrate cancer cells. ANNALS OF NEW YORK ACADEMY OF SCIENCES 1031: 391-394; Conte E, Floridi A, Aisa C, et al. (2004).

Genotoxicity of Naturally Occuring Hydroxyanthraquinones; Johannes Westendorf, Hildegard Marquaradt, Barbara Poginsky, Marion Dominaik, Juergen Schmidt & Hans Marquardt.

Glycosylation and rheumatic disease Proceedings of the Royal Society of Medicine's 5th Jenner Symposium, Axford J.S.

HPLC Analysis of Aloe – A Guarantee of Top Quality; Ronald P. Pelley, Ph.D., M.D.

Green tea and cancer chemoprevention. Mutation Res. 1999; 428:339-344; Suganuma M, Okabe S, Sueoka N, et al.

Green tea and skin -- anticarcinogenic effects. J Invest Dermatol. 1994; 102:3-7; Mukhtar H, Katiyar SK, Agarwal R.

Green tea and thermogenesis: interactions between catechin-polyphenols, caffeine and sympathetic activity. Int J Obes Relat Metab Disord. 2000; 24:252-258; Dulloo AG, Seydoux J, Girardier L, et al.

Green tea compounds inhibit tyrosine phosphorylation of PDGF beta-receptor and transformation of A172 human glioblastoma. FEBS Lett. 2000; 471:51-55; Sachinidis A, Seul C, Seewald S, et al.

Green tea polyphenols and cancer: biologic mechanisms and practical implications. Nutr Rev. 1999; 57:78-83; Ahmad N, Mukhtar H.

Green tea polyphenols (flavan 3-ols) prevent oxidative modification of low density lipoproteins: an ex vivo study in humans. J Nutr Biochem. 2000; 11:216-222; Miura Y, Chiba T, Miura S, et al.

Harper's, Illustrated Biochemistry, 27th Edition, page 424-42, 436, 464, 618.

How Do They Grow Aloe? (Farm & Ranch Magazine).

How the Immune System Develops; Irving L. Weissman & Max D. Cooper.

How the Immune System Recognized Invaders; Charles A. Janeway, Jr.

How the Immune System Recognizes the Body; Phillippa Marrack & John W. Kappler.

Hydrogen Peroxide Metabolism in Human Monocytes During Differentiation in Vitro; Akira Nakagawara, Carl F. Nathan & Zanvil A. Cohn.

IASC Certification Healing Old Credibility Wounds (Aloe Today, Winter 1992 – Todd Waller).

Identification of Some Prostanoids in Aloe Vera Extracts; M. Afzal.

Immunological Consequences of UV-B Radiation; Margaret L. Kripke.

Immunological Effects of Ultraviolet Radiation; Margaret L. Kripke.

Immunology and Photocarcinogenesis; Margaret L. Kripke.

Immunoreactive Lectins in Leaf Gel From Aloe Barbadensis Miller; Wendell D. Winters.

Immunosuppressive Effect of Emodin, A Free Radical Generator; Huei-Chen Huang, Jin-Hsia Chang, Shiu-Feng Tung, Rong-Tsun Wu, Marie L. Foegh & Shu-Hsun Chu.

Impaired Immune Function in Patients with Xeroderma Pigmentosum; Margaret L. Kripke, Warwick L. Morison, Cora Bucana, Nemat Hashem, James E. Cleaver & James L. German.

Identification of (-)-epicatechin metabolites and their metabolic fate in the rat. Drug Metab Disp. 1999; 27:309-316; Okushio K, Suzuki M, Matsumoto N, et al.

Induction of Bax and activation of caspases during beta-sitosterol-mediated apoptosis in human colon cancer cells. Int J Oncol. 2003;23(6):1657-1662. (PubMed); Choi YH, Kong KR, Kim YA, et al.

Infectious Diabetes; D. Kaufman and D. Holland, M.D.

Infectious Diseases & The Immune System; William E. Paul.

Influence of a cod liver oil diet in diabetics type 1 on fatty acid patterns and platelet aggregation. Biomed.Biochim.Acta 1984; 43:S351-S353; Schimke E, Hildebrandt R, Beitz J et al.

Influence of a cod liver oil diet in healthy and insulin-dependent diabetic volunteers on fatty acid pattern, inhibition of prostacyclin formation by low density lipoprotein (LDL) and platelet thromboxane. Klin.Wochenschr. 1986; 64:793-9; Beitz J, Schimke E, Liebaug U et al.

Inhibition of Arachidonic Acid Oxidation In Vitro by Vehicle Components; Neal S. Penneys.

Inhibition Of Aids Virus Replication By Acemannan In Vitro; Kahlon et al, 1991.

Inhibition of UV-Induced Immune Suppression and Interleukin-10 Production by Plant Oligosaccharides and Polysaccharides; Faith Strickland, Alan Darvill, Peter Albersheim, Stefab Ebergardm, Narcys Oaykt & Ronald Pelley.

Inhibitory effect of Chinese green tea on endothelial cell-induced LDL oxidation. Atherosclerosis. 2000; 148:67-73; Yang TTC, Koo MWL.

Inside Aloe Vera (Optimal Health Journal, Vol. 1, issue 4).

Internal Uses of Aloe Vera; Ivan E. Danhof, M.D., Ph.D., North Texas Medical Association.

Interview with Dr. Robert Picker, M.D., Public Scrutiny, May 1982, Vol. XXVII, No. 11.

Isolation and Characterization of the Glycoprotein Fraction with a Proliferation-Promoting Activty on Human and Hamster Cells in Vitro from Aloe Vera Gel; Akira Yagi, Taro Egusa, Mami Arase, Miyo Tanabe, Hiroshi Tsuji.

Isolation & Structure Analysis of a Glucomannan from the Leaves of Aloe Arborescens var. Miller; Thomas Woznicwski, Wolfgang Blaschek & Gerhard Franz.

Kids Who Shun Veggies Risk III Health Later (USA Today – Tim Friend).

Life Extension, March 2007

Long-term effect of eicosapentaenoic acid ethyl (EPA-E) on albuminuria of non-insulin dependent diabetic patients. Diabetes Res.Clin Pract. 1995; 28:35-40; Shimizu H, Ohtani K, Tanaka Y, Sato N, Mori M, Shimomura Y.

Lycopene as the most efficient biological carotenoid singlet oxygen quencher. Arch. Biochem. Biophys., 274:532-538; Di Mascio, P., Kaiser, S., and Sies, H. (1989)

Matrix metalloproteinase inhibition by green tea catechins. Biochim Biophys Acta. 2000; 1478:51-60; Demeule M, Brossard M, Pagé, M, et al.

Mechanism of Anti-Inflammatory & Anti-Thermal Burn action of Aloe Arborescens Mill. Var. Natalensis Berger; Masafumi Obata, Shosuke Ito, Hidehiko Beppu & Keisuke Fujita.

Meta-analysis: the effect of probiotic administration on antibiotic-associated diarrhea. Ailment Pharmacol Ther. 2002; 16: 1461-1467 Entrez PubMed 12182746, Cremonini F, Di Caro S, Nista EC, Bartolozzi F, Capelli G, Gasbarrini G, Gasbarrini A.

Mineral Analyses of Vegetarian, Health, and Conventional Foods: Magnesium, Zinc, Copper and Manganese Content; Deborah A. McNeill, Perveen S. Ali & Young S. Song.

Modern Nutrition in Health and Disease. 8th ed. Philadelphia, PA: Lea and Febiger, 1994:326-41; Farrell P and Roberts R. Vitamin E. In: Shils M, Olson JA, and Shike M, ed.

Modern Nutrition in Health and Disease. 10th ed. Baltimore: Williams & Wilkins, 1999:347-62; Traber MG. Vitamin E. In: Shils ME, Olson JA, Shike M, Ross AC, ed.

Molecular Biology of the Cell. 3d ed. New York: Garland, 2002; Alberts, Bruce, et al.

Morphology & Anatomy in Aloinae. I Gasteria Verrucosa (Mill) Haworth; Mogens Wellendorf.

Multiparameter Analysis of Aloe Barbadensis Gel Extracts; Ronald P. Pelley, Ph.D., M.D.

[Multiple actions of EGCG, the main component of green tea]. [Article in French]. Bull Cancer. 1999; 86:721-724; L'Allemain G.

My Favorite Plant Aloe Vera; Gayle Gates.

Myth, Magic, Witchcraft or Fact? Aloe Vera Revisited; John P. Heggers Martin C. Robson.

Natural sources of carotenoids from plants and oils. Meth. Enzymol., 213: 142-167; Ong, A.S.H., and E.S. Tee. (1992).

"Neuroprotective properties of the natural vitamin E alpha-tocotrienol." Stroke 36 (10): 2258-64. PMID 16166580; Khanna S, Roy S, Slivka A, Craft T, Chaki S, Rink C, Notestine M, DeVries A, Parinandi N, Sen C (2005).

New carotenoids: recent progress. Invited Lecture 2. Abstracts of the 12th International Carotenoid Symposium, Cairns, Australia, July 1999; Mercadante, A. (1999).

New Uses for Aloe Vera (Natural Health Magazine – Karen Barr).

"Nutrient Receptors and Gene Expression." In Nutrition and Gene Expression, edited by Carolyn D. Berdanier and James L. Hargrove. Boca

Raton, Fla.: CRC Press, 1993; Berdanier, Carolyn D., and James L. Hargrove.

Panacea or Old Wives' Tales? Ellis G. Bovik, D.D.S., M.S.D.

Partial normalization by dietary cod liver oil of increased microvascular albumin leakage in patients with insulin-dependent diabetes and albuminuria. N.Engl.J Med. 1989;321:1572-7; Jensen T, Stender S, Goldstein K, Holmer G, Deckert T.

Partial Purification and Some Properties of an Antibacterial Compound from Aloe Vera; Hadassa Levin, R. Hazenfratz, J. Friedman, D. Palevitch & M. Perl.

Pharmacological Studies on a Plant Lectin, Aloctin A.I. Growth inhibition of Mouse Methyl.

Plasma concentration of carotenoids after large doses of beta-carotene. Am. J. Clin. Nutr., Sep 52:3, 500-1; Mathews-Roth, MM. (1990).

Polypeptides of Aloe Barbadensis Miller, Effects of Aloe Extracts of Human Normal and Tumor Cells, Immunoreactive Lectins in Leaf gel From Aloe Barbadensis Miller, S. L. Udupa, A. L. Udupa & D. R. Kulkarni.cholanthrene-Induced Fibrosarcoma: K. Imanishi, T. Ishiguro, H. Saito & I. Suzuki.

Polypeptides of Aloe Barbadensis Miller; Dr. Wendell Winters & Pamela B. Yang.

"Post-Transcriptional Control via Iron-Responsive Elements: The Impact of Aberrations in Hereditary Disease." Mutation Research 437 (1999): 219–230; Mikulits, Wolfgang, Matthias Schranzhofer, Hartmut Beug, and Ernst W. Müllner.

Potential Benefits from Orally-ingested internal Aloe Vera Gel; Ivan E. Danhoff, Ph.D., M.D.

"Potential Mechanisms of Metabolic Imprinting that Lead to Chronic Disease." American Journal of Clinical Nutrition 69 (1999): 179–197; Waterland, Robert A., and Cutberto Garza.

Potential uses of probiotics in clinical practice. Clin Microbiol Rev. 2003; 16:658-72. Entrez PubMed 14557292, Reid G, Jass J, Sebulsky MT, McCormick JK.

Prevalence, severity, and comorbidity of twelve-month DSM-IV disorders in the National Comorbidity Survey Replication (NCS-R). Archives of General Psychiatry, 2005 Jun;62(6):617-27; Kessler RC, Chiu WT, Demler O, Walters EE.

Prevention of Atheromateous Heart Disease,1985 Aloe's blood glucose lowering, cholesterol and triglyceride lowering effects, O.P. Agarwal, M.D., F.I.C.A., Uttar Pradesh, India: Angiology; Volume 36, Number 8, August 1985 – The Journal of Vascular Diseases Published twelve times a year under the auspices of Westminster Publications, Inc.

Prevention of collagen-induced arthritis in mice by a polyphenolic fraction from green tea. Proc Natl Acad Sci USA. 1999; 96:4524-4529; Haqqi TM, Anthony DD, Gupta S, et al.

Principles of Wound Healing and Growth Factor Considerations; Stephen J. Skokan, B.S. & Robert H. Davis, Ph.D.

Probiotics an overview of beneficial effects. Antonie Van Leeuwenhoek. 2002; 82:279-89. Entrez PubMed 12369194, Ouwehand AC, Salminen S, Isolauri E.

Probiotics and prevention of atopic disease: 4-year follow-up of a randomized placebo-controlled trial Lancet. 2003; 361:1869-1871. Entrez PubMed 12788576, Kalliomaki M, Salminen S, Poussa T, Arvilommi H, Isolauri E.

Probiotic bacteria in the management of atopic disease: underscoring the importance of viability. J Pediatr Gastroenterol Nutr. 2003; 36:223-227 Entrez PubMed 12548058, Kirjavainen PV, Salminen SJ, Isolauri E.

Probiotic lactobacilli: an innovative tool to correct the malabsorption syndrome of vegetarians? Med Hypotheses. 2005; 65(6):1132-5. Entrez PubMed 16095846, Famularo G, De Simone C, Pandey V, Sahu AR, Minisola G.

Processed Aloe Vera Administered Topically Inhibits Inflammation; Gregory A. Rouw.

Prostaglandins & Thromboxane; John P. Heggers & Martin C. Robson.

Prostanoid Derivatives in Thermal Injury; John P. Heggers & Martin C. Robson.

Prostate cancer chemoprevention by green tea. Semin Urol Oncol. 1999; 17:70-76; Gupta S, Ahmad N, Mukhtar H.

Purification & Characterization of a Gliuthathione Peroxidase from theAloe Vera Plant; F. Sabeh, T. Wright & S.J. Norton.

Purification & Characterization of Two Lectins from Aloe Arborescens Mill; Ikuo Suzuki, Hiroko Saito, Shigeki Inoue, Shunsuke Migita & Taijo Takahashi.

Purification of a Glutathione Peroxidase from the Aloe Vera Plant, F. Sabeh, T. Wright, & S. J. Norton.

Race is on to Develop Sugar-Based Anti-inflammatory, Antitumor Drugs; Stu Borman.

Reduced Gluthathione as an Effector of Phosphoenolpyruvate Carboxylase of the Crassulacean Acid Metabolism Plant Sedum Praealtum D.C.; Yiannis Manetas and Nikos A. Gavalas.

Retardation of the Ageing Process in Rats by Food Restriction, B. P. Yu, E.J. Masoro, I. Shimokawa .

Reversal of UVB-Induced Suppression of Contact Sensitivity in C3H Mice by Topical Administration of Aloe Barbadensis Gel Extracts; Faith Strickland, Ronald Pelley, Donald Hill & Margaret Kripke.

Roentgen Dermatitis Treated with Fresh Whole Leaf Aloe Vera; C.F. Collins, D.D.S., M.D. & Creston Collins, M.S.
Say Aloe to an Age Old Remedy (Fort Worth Star Telegram).

Scientist Helps Hasten the Healing of Young and Old (Fort Worth Star – Steve Gariepy).

Screening of Natural Sources for Antiinflammatory Activity (Review); B. Sener & F. Bingol.

Secrets of Long Life, New York, Devin-Adair Publishers, 1993; Walker, Morton.

Skin Cancer Cases Climbing, Experts Say (The Dallas Morning News – Laura Bell).

Skin Penetration of Mucilage and Aloe Vera; Robert H. Davis, Ph.D.

Some External Uses of Aloe; Ivan E. Danhof, Ph.D., M.D.

Some Sunscreens may be ineffective, Study Finds (Chicago Tribune – Jan. 19, 1994 – Scripps Howard).

Soothing Succulent Aloe Vera (Texas Highway Magazine, Janet Edwards, Jan. 98).

Stabilized Aloe Vera: Effect on Human Skin Cells; Ivan E. Danhof Ph.D., M.D. & Bill H. McAnnaley, Ph.D.

Sterol transporters: targets of natural sterols and new lipid lowering drugs. Pharmacol Ther. 2005; 105(3):333-341. (PubMed) ; Sudhop T, Lutjohann D, von Bergmann K.

Stimulation of Neuron-like Cell Growth by Aloe Substances; Dr. Wendell Winters, Catherine Bouther, Virgil Schirf.

Stimulation of Primary Rate Hepatocytes; Hans Marquardt.

Structure and properties of carotenoids in relation to function. FASEB J., 9:1551-1558; Britton, G. (1995).

Structure Determination of Polysaccharides in Aloe Arborescens var. Natalensis; Akira Yagi, Hiroshi Nishimura, Takao Shida & Itsu Nishioka.

Structure of the D-Galactan Isolated from Aloe Barbadensis Miller; Gaurhai Mandal & Amalendu Das.

Structure of the Glucomannan Isolated From The Leaves of Aloe Barbadensis Miller; Gaurhai Mandal & Amalendu Das.

Structural identification of two metabolites of catechins and their kinetics in human urine and blood after tea ingestion. Chem Res Toxicol. 2000; 13:177-184; Li C, Lee M-J, Sheng S, et al.

Structural Studies of Polysaccharides from Aloe Vera; D. Channe Gowda, Belkavadi Neelisiddaiah & Yernool V. Anjaneyalu.

Structural Studies of the Glucomannan from Aloe Vahombe; Farhad Radjabi, Claudine Amar & Erna Vilkas.

Structural Studies of the Polysaccharide from Aloe Plicatilis Miller; Berit Smestad Paulsen, Egil Fagerheim & Elna Overbye.

Structural Study of an Acidic Polysaccharide Isolated From Aloe Arborescens Mill. I. Periodate Oxidation & Partial Acid Hydrolysis; Mirjana Hranisavljevic-Jakovljevic & Jelena Miljkovic-Stojanovic.

Studies on Alysis of Organic Acids & Amino Acids in Various Aloe Species; Masaaki Ishikawa, Masatoshi Yamamoto & Toshio Masui.

Studies on Glucogalactomannan from the Leaves of Aloe Vera Tourn. (EX.LINN.); Q.N. Hag and A. Hannan.

Studies on the Constituents of Aloe Arborescens Mill. Var. Natalensis Berger. I. The Structures of Two New Aleosin Esters; Kenji Makino, Akira Yagi & Itsuo Nishioka.

Studies on the Constituents of Aloe Arborescens Mill. Var. Natalensis Berger. II. The Structures of Two New Aleosin Esters; Kenji Makino, Akira Yagi & Itsuo Nishioka.

Study Shows Aloe Prolongs Life, Decreases Incidence of Disease (Nexus May/June 1997).

Sugar Composition in Macromolecular Fraction from Aloe Vera; Akira Yagi.

Sun and Ultraviolet Ray Exposure; Margaret L. Kripke.

Targeted Delivery of Superoxide Dismutase to Macrophages Via Mannose Receptor-Mediated Mechanism, Yoshinobu Takakura, Sada Masuda, Hikeaki Tokuda, Makiya Nishikawa & Mitsuru Hashida.

Tea catechin supplementation increases antioxidant capacity and prevents phospholipid hydroperoxidation in plasma of humans. J Agric Food Chem. 1999; 47:3967-3973; Nakagawa K, Ninomiya M, Okubo T, et al.

The Aloe Alternative; Bruce Magness.

The Aloe Vera Phenomenon: A review of the Properties and Modern Uses of the Leaf Parenchyma Gel; Douglas Grindlay & T. Reynolds.

The Art and Science of Burn Care; John A. Boswick, Jr., MD, FACS.

The Compounds in Aloe Leaf Exudates: A Review; T. Reynolds.

The Conductor-Orchestra Concept of Aloe Vera; Robert H. Davis, Ph.D., Scientific Advisor and Research Consultant, Aloecorp, Professor Emeritus of Physiology, Pennsylvania College of Podiatric Medicine.

The Current Status of Aloe Vera Research; William B. Bowles.

The Drug Aloes of Commerce, With Special Reference to the Cape Species; W.H. Hodge.

The Efficacy of the Aloe Plants Chemical Constituents and Biological Activities; Takayuki Suga, Toshifumi Hirata.

The Evaluation of Natural Substances in the Treatment of Adjuvant Arthritis; Denice C. Hanley, William A.B. Solomon, Barry Saffran & Robert H. Davis, Ph.D.

The Evolution of Aloes: New Clues from their Leaf Chemistry; AM Cviljoen & B-E van Wyk.

The External Use of Aloes, J.E. Crewe, M.D.

The Glucomannan Sytem From Aloe Vahombe (Lilliaceae). III. Comparative Studies on the Glucomannan Components Isolated from the Leaves; Erna Vilkas & Farhad Radjabi-Nassab.

The Healing Power of the Aloe Vera (New Women Magazine – Bargyla Ratceaver, Ph.D.).

The How, Where, and What of Good Aloe, Dr. Reginald McDaniel.

The Immune System as a Therapeutic Agent; Hans Wigzell.

The Immunology of Skin Cancer; Margaret L. Kripke.

The Isolation of an Active Inhibitory System from an Extract of Aloe Vera; Robert H. Davis, Ph.D., William L. Parker, B.A., Richard T. Samson, B.S. & Douglas P. Murdoch, B.S., Kenneth Y. Rosenthal, Linda R. Cesario.

"The Role of Orphan Nuclear Receptors in the Regulation of Cholesterol Homeostasis." Annual Review of Cellular and Developmental Biology 16 (2000): 459–481; Repa, Joyce J., and David J. Mangelsdorf.

The role of probiotics in the treatment and prevention of Helicobacter pylori infection. Int J Antimicrob Agents. 2003; 22:360-366. Entrez PubMed 14522098, Hamilton-Miller JM.

The Role of Topical Agents in the Healing of Full Thickness Wounds; Melissa A. Watcher, M.D., Ronald G. Wheeland, M.D.

The Soothing Aloe Vera Plant (Delicious Magazine, Sept. 1997 – Sue Woodard).

The Stimulation of Postdermabrasion Wound Healing with Stabilized Aloe Vera Gel-Polyethylene Oxide Dressing; James E. Fulton, Jr., M.D., Ph.D.

The Therapeutic Efficacy of Aloe Vera Cream (Dermaide Aloe) in Thermal Injuries: Two Case Reports; Lee M. Cera, John P. Heggers, Martin C. Robson, William J. Hagstrom.

The World Health Organization. The World Health Report 2004: Changing History, Annex Table 3: Burden of disease in DALYs by cause, sex, and mortality stratum in WHO regions, estimates for 2002. Geneva: WHO, 2004.

Therapeutic Protocol for Thermally Injured Animals & its Successful Use in an Extensively Burned Rhesus Monkey; Lee M. Cera, John P. Heggers, William J. Hagstrom & Martin C. Robson.

Therapy & Treatment with Aloe Vera; Frank Murray.

Three Chromone Components from Aloe Vera Leaves; Nobuyuki Okamura, Noriko Hine, Toshihiro Fujioka, Kunihide.

Tissue Culture of Aloe Arborescens Miller var. Natalensis Berger; Kaoru Kawai, Hidehiko Beppu, Takaaki Koike & Keisuke Fujita.

Tocotrienol-rich fraction from palm oil and gene expression in human breast cancer cells. ANNALS OF THE NEW YORK ACADEMY OF SCIENCES 1031: 143-157; Nesaretnam K, Ambra R, Selvaduray KR, et al. (2004).

Topical Anti-Inflammatory Activity of Aloe Vera as Measured by Ear Swelling; Robert H. Davis, Mark G. Leitner, Joseph M. Russo.

Topical Effect of Aloe with Ribonucleic Acid and Vitamin C on Adjuvant Arthritis; Robert H. Davis, Ph.D., Eugene Shapiro, Patrick S. Agnew.

Treating Injuries with Aloe Vera (Runners World/Jan. 1993 – Chuck Piper w/Kevin Baxter).

Two Functionally and Chemically Distinct Immunomodulatory Compounds in the Gel of Aloe Vera , L.A. T Hart, Van Enckevort, H. van Dijk, R. Zaat, K. de Silva & R.P. van Dijk.

Use of cod liver oil during pregnancy associated with lower risk of Type I diabetes in the offspring. Diabetologia 2000; 43:1093-8; Stene LC, Ulriksen J, Magnus P, Joner G.

U.S. scientists extend the life of human cells, British Medical Journal, Jan, 1998

U.S. Department of Agriculture, Agricultural Research Service. 2004. USDA National Nutrient Database for Standard Reference, Release 16-1. Nutrient Data Laboratory Home.

Uses of Aloe in Treating Leg Ulcers and Dermatoses; M. El Zawahry, M.D., M. Rashad Hegazy, M.D. & M. Helal, B.Ph.

Vasorelaxants from Chinese Herbs, Emodin and Scoparone, Possess Immunosuppressive Properties; Huei-Chen Huang, Shu-Hsun Chu & Pei-Dawn Lee Chao.

Vitamin A as "anti-infective" therapy, 1920-1940. J Nutr 1999; 129:783-91; Semba RD.

Vitamin E: Beyond antioxidant function. Am J Clin Nutr 1995; 62:1501S-9S; Traber MG and Packer L.

Why drinking green tea could prevent cancer. Nature. 1997; 387:561; Jankun J, Selman SH, Swiercz R, Skrzypczak-Jankun E.

Wound Healing – Oral and Topical Activity of Aloe Vera; Robert H. Davis, Ph.D. Mark G. Leitner, RPh, DPM, Joseph M. Russo, DPM & Megan E. Byrne, B.S.

Wound Healing Potential of Aloe and Other Chemotherapeutic Agents; John P. Heggers, Ahmet Kucukcelebi, Catherine J. Stabenau, Francis Ko, Lyle D. Broemeling, Wendell Winters, Catherine Bouthet and Martin C. Robson.